1500 QUESTIONS FOR THE DCH/ MRCPCH FOUNDATION OF PRACTICE EXAM

Dr. Farah Alam –Mirza MRCGP, DCH, DRCOG, DFSRH, MBBS, Postgraduate Certificate for Teachers in Primary Care

General Practitioner
London

Copyright 2016 © Dr. Farah Alam –Mirza

All rights reserved. No part of this publication may be reproduced, stored in a retrieval system, or transmitted, in any form or by any means, electronic, mechanical, photocopying, recording or otherwise without the prior permission of the copyright owner.

ISBN 13 978 1502822932

ISBN 10 1502822938

The information contained within this book was obtained by the author from reliable sources. However, while every effort has been made to ensure its accuracy; no responsibility for loss, damage or injury occurring to any person acting or refraining from action as a result of information contained herein can be accepted by the publishers or author.

CONTENTS

Preface

QUESTIONS

Paper 1..6

Paper 2...30

Paper 3...54

Paper 4...77

Paper 5..100

ANSWERS

Answers Paper 1......................................125

Answers Paper 2......................................155

Answers Paper 3......................................180

Answers Paper 4......................................205

Answers Paper 5......................................227

Bibliography..248

Index..250

Preface

The principal aim of this book is to provide a rigorous and challenging set of practice questions for candidates to revise and prepare for the MRCPCH Foundation of Practice exam, and will prove a useful tool for preparation for the Diploma of Child Health. It is divided into five practice papers containing sixty stems with five multiple-choice true/false questions each. Detailed explanations of the answers have been provided to aid understanding and knowledge. This will be an invaluable asset to candidates aiming to reach the standard required for core specialist training, and for general practitioners with a special interest in paediatrics.

QUESTIONS

Multiple Choice Questions- Paper 1

Decide whether each statement (A-E) is true or false.

1. Anorexia nervosa may cause:

A. Fungal skin infections

B. Increased metabolic rate

C. Hypokalaemia

D. Reduced cortisol

E. Increased thyroxine

2. Investigating congenital heart disease:

A. Pulmonary oedema may be evident on chest x-ray in atrial septal defect

B. Cardiomegaly is seen on chest x-ray in more than 60% of children with large ventricular- septal defects

C. Pulmonary plethora is seen on chest x-ray in a Tetralogy of Fallot

D. Right bundle branch block may be seen on ECG in atrial septal defect in the lead V1

E. Rib notching may be seen on chest x-ray in coarctation of the aorta

3. Fears and phobias in childhood:

A. Separation anxiety from 10 months

B. Stranger anxiety from six months

C. School phobia is common in social class III and IV

D. Fear of nightmares up to 11 years

E. One third of children with school phobia will have adult neuroses

4. Bronchiectasis:

A. Is associated with hypergammaglobulinaemia

B. May occur after a foreign body inhalation

C. May occur with measles

D. Cyanosis may be present in severe cases

E. Can occur after childhood pneumonia

5. Cystic fibrosis:

A. Is associated with nasal polyps

B. Diabetes is found in 50% of teenage cases

C. Neonatal screening is available

D. One in 2000 live births is affected

E. Asthma coexists in 50%

6. Side effects of methylphenidate include:

A. Weight gain

B. Insomnia

C. Tics

D. Psychosis

E. Lowers seizure threshold

7. Child abuse:

A. Neglect is the commonest form

B. Mortality is 500 children per year in England

C. One in 1000 children suffer severe physical abuse in Britain

D. Girls are more likely to be on the child protection register up to the age of 10

E. Sexual abuse often begins over five years of age

8. Skeletal survey should be done in the following:

A. Physical abuse in a child over three years

B. Severe soft tissue injury in an older child

C. Non-accidental injuries for example, fractures

D. Coma

E. Child dying in suspicious or unusual circumstances

9. Prolonged QT syndrome:

A. Usually presents in late teens

B. Prolonged if QTc is greater than 440 ms

C. Associated with syncope during exercise, stress or emotion

D. Associated with Cisapride

E. Associated with Omeprazole

10. Orders under the Children's Act 1989:

A. Police protection order lasts for 48 hours

B. Emergency protection order lasts for eight days

C. Emergency protection order is issued by the court

D. Child assessment order lasts for three days

E. Supervision order lasts for six months.

11. The social services Child protection process:

A. Strategy meeting should take place within seven days

B. Initial child protection case conference should be held within fifteen working days of the strategy meeting

C. Initial child protection case conference should be within 42 days of case referral

D. The child is placed on the child protection register at the strategy meeting

E. Child protection review is carried out yearly

12. Cystic fibrosis may present with:

A. Meconium ileus

B. Obstructive jaundice

C. Steatorrhoea

D. Anaemia

E. Female infertility

13. Snoring:

A. If severe may lead to pulmonary hypertension and cor pulmonale

B. May lead to poor growth

C. Is seen in Pierre- Robin sequence

D. Is abnormal if associated with obstructive apnoea

E. Common in children with Down's syndrome

14. Causes of a long PR interval (more than 0.16 s) are:

A. Atrial septal defect

B. Myocarditis

C. Digoxin toxicity

D. Hypokalaemia

E. Wolff- Parkinson- White syndrome

15. Regarding whooping cough:

A. It is rare in the UK

B. Incubation period is 14 to 21 days

C. Associated with high mortality

D. Culture is from nasal swab

E. Lymphocytopenia is seen on blood film

16. Cerebral palsy:

A. In diplegia the arms are more affected than the legs

B. Hand preference at eight months is normal

C. In hemiplegia the predominant sign is that the affected limb is flaccid and hypotonic

D. Quadriplegia is often associated with intellectual impairment

E. In quadriplegia the birth history is usually normal

17. Epidemiology:

A. Incidence is the proportion of a defined group having a disease at any one time

B. Prevalence is the proportion of a defined group developing a disease within a stated period

C. 40% of all childhood deaths occur in the first year in England and Wales

D. Prevalence is useful when measuring chronic conditions

E. Incidents measures the rate of occurrence of new cases

18. Mortality rates:

A. Stillbirth rate is the number of infants born dead with the gestational age of 24 weeks per 1000 births

B. Perinatal mortality rate is the number of stillbirths and deaths during the first 28 days of life per 1000 total births

C. Early neonatal mortality rate is the number of deaths at up to 6 days of life per 1000 total births

D. Neonatal mortality rate is the number of deaths up to 28 days of life per 1000 total births

E. Infant mortality rate is the number of deaths in infants under one year per 1000 live births

19. Mortality rates:

A. A major cause of neonatal mortality is pre-maturity

B. Major causes of infant mortality are perinatal problems associated with pre-maturity and congenital anomalies

C. After one year of age, injury and poisoning are the major causes of death

D. Mortality rates are lower for boys

E. Mortality rates are higher in social class I and 2

20. Statistics:

A. Cross-sectional studies determine the incidence of a certain condition

B. Cohort studies give estimation of incidence

C. Cohort studies are useful for studying rare diseases

D. Case-control studies are particularly prone to bias

E. Case-control studies are useful for studying rare diseases

21. Screening tests:

A. Sensitivity is the number of people without the condition who are correctly identified by the test

B. Specificity is the number of people with the condition who are correctly identified by the test

C. Positive predictive value is the number of positive screening results that are correct

D. The predictive value of a positive result falls as the prevalence rises

E. Low specificity leads to lots of false positives and cost implications

22. Haemophilus influenza B (Hib) vaccine:

A. Is a live vaccine

B. Full course is required if over one year old and not immune

C. Routine immunisation is recommended up to 4 years

D. H. Influenza B infection may cause cellulitis, pericarditis and septic arthritis

E. Is contraindicated if there is a history of prolonged jaundice

23. Regarding Measles, Mumps and Rubella:

A. Mumps may cause pancreatitis

B. Rubella may cause arthritis and arthralgia in adults

C. Sub-acute sclerosing pan-encephalitis (SSPE) may occur seven years after measles infection

D. There is a 20% failure rate from primary vaccination with MMR at 12 to 18 months of age

E. Rubella infection peaks in the 1 to 4 year age group

24. Adverse reactions to the MMR vaccine include:

A. Rash after a week

B. Parotid swelling after two weeks

C. Encephalopathy

D. Idiopathic thrombocytopenic purpura

E. Arthropathy

25. Hepatitis B immunisation:

A. Infants born to mothers who are Hepatitis B surface antigen (HbsAg) positive and anti-HBe positive have vaccine and immunoglobulin at birth

B. If the mother is HbsAg positive and HBe Ag positive the baby receives vaccine only

C. Further doses are recommended at one month, two months and 12 months of age

D. HbsAg testing is carried out at 15 months of age

E. Booster vaccine is given at five years of age

26. Visual loss:

A. Visual impairment is defined as corrected acuity of less than 6/18 in the better eye

B. Visual impairment may not be correctable after three years of age

C. In Amblyopia, the defect is not correctable by glasses

D. About 20% of cases are of genetic origin

E. The defect is most commonly in the retina

27. Squint:

A. Prevalence is about 10%

B. The cover test is performed at 100 cm

C. In a latent squint there is movement of the uncovered eye on covering

D. In a manifest squint there is movement of the covered eye on uncovering

E. Alternating squints have good prognosis

28. Hearing loss:

A. Prevalence of congenital sensorineural hearing loss is 4 to 11 in 100

B. Pendred's syndrome is associated with conductive hearing loss

C. Due to middle ear disease may produce a conductive hearing loss of 30 dB

D. Stay of upto 12 hours in the neonatal intensive care unit increases the risk of hearing loss

E. Treacher- Collins syndrome is associated with conductive hearing loss

29. Hearing screening:

A. Neonatal screening with evoked otoacoustic emissions checks the cochlear pathways only

B. Distraction test is done at 7 to 9 months

C. The co-operative language test is done at four years of age

D. 50 dB is required for normal speech to develop

E. The school sweep test is performed with a free field audio meter

30. Behavioural problems:

A. Are associated with high parental IQ

B. Are seen in children in high-rise housing

C. Marital discord leads to externalising behaviour in girls

D. Girls are less vulnerable than boys

E. Are commoner in children with low IQ

31. Tuberous sclerosis:

A. More than 50% of cases are sporadic

B. May present with infantile spasms

C. 20% have renal involvement

D. Adenoma sebaceum over the nose and cheeks is seen in 50% by five years

E. Epilepsy is present in 50%

32. Neurofibromatosis:

A. Type II may present in the second decade

B. Type I is associated with an increased incidence of Wilm's tumour

C. Type I is associated with congenital buphthalmos

D. Type I accounts for 10% of cases

E. Lisch nodules are a feature in Type II

33. Tuberous sclerosis:

A. Incidence is approximately 1 in 100,000

B. Gene is located on chromosome 7

C. Intracranial calcification is seen in 10%

D. Amelanotic naevi needing Wood's light to see may be present

E. Retinal phacomata may be seen near the optic disc

34. Inguinal hernias and hydrocoeles:

A. Inguinal hernias are present in 9 to 11% of preterm babies

B. 15% are bilateral

C. Referral for surgery is necessary for all inguinal hernias

D. Hydrocoeles should be operated on by 12 months of age

E. A hydrocoele may be associated with a tumour

35. Prader-Willi syndrome is associated with:

A. Obesity

B. Failure to thrive in infancy

C. Absence of maternal contribution to chromosome 15

D. Undescended testes and cryptorchidism

E. Tall stature

36. Prader-Willi syndrome is associated with:

A. Hypotonia in infancy

B. Diabetes mellitus

C. Breech presentation at birth

D. Severe mental retardation

E. Inappropriate laughter

37. Phimosis and paraphimosis:

A. Phimosis is common below five years

B. Paraphimosis is a surgical emergency

C. Phimosis needs follow-up

D. Children with Balanitis Xerotica Obliterans (BXO) need a surgical opinion

E. 1% of 17-year-olds have non-retractile foreskins

38. Acute scrotum in childhood:

A. Orchitis is commoner in post-pubertal boys.

B. Torsion of the testis is most frequent at 10 to 12 years of age

C. Torsion of the appendix testis leads to an increased risk of testicular torsion

D. Idiopathic scrotal oedema is commonest in 1 to 3-year-olds

E. Idiopathic scrotal oedema may spread beyond the scrotum and is very painful and tender

39. Pyloric stenosis:

A. Incidence is 2 in 1000 live births

B. Commonly presents at 4 to 6 months of age

C. There may be a genetic component in aetiology

D. Bilious vomiting is a common feature

E. Constipation is common

40. Intussusception:

A. Commonly occurs in girls

B. Peaks at 5 to 9 months of age

C. Vomiting may be bilious

D. Fever is common

E. Perforation of the colon during hydrostatic reduction is common

41. Spina bifida:

A. Most commonly occurs at L5 and S1

B. Myelomeningocoeles account for 10% of overt spina bifida

C. In a meningocoele, there is usually abnormal neurology

D. Hydrocephalus is rare in a meningocoele

E. May be associated with precocious puberty

42. Spina bifida:

A. Strabismus may be present

B. Hydrocephalus is commonly present due to Arnold – Chiari malformation

C. Can be diagnosed antenatally

D. There may be associated kyphoscoliosis

E. Vesicoureteric reflux is common and may require surgery

43. Noonan's syndrome:

A. Is associated with severe mental retardation

B. Congenital cardiac defects are present in 20%

C. Low set ears

D. Ovarian dysgenesis

E. There may be feeding problems in the neonatal period

44. Pierre- Robin sequence:

A. Sporadic inheritance

B. May result in airway obstruction

C. Is associated with reduced movements in- utero

D. There is maxillary hypoplasia

E. High- arched palate

45. Cerebral palsy:

A. 15% of cerebral palsy is due to perinatal causes

B. Epilepsy is present in 25% with spastic diplegia

C. Mental retardation may be present in 18 to 50% of children with hemiplegia

D. Strabismus is common in hemiplegia

E. There may be cystic softening in the region of the middle cerebral artery

46. Cerebral palsy:

A. There may be involvement of the bulbar muscles in spastic quadriplegia

B. Spastic quadriplegia is associated with damage to the brain stem

C. Babies may be small for dates

D. Intelligence is usually impaired in the dyskinetic group

E. The overall incidence of cerebral palsy has increased in the last 20 years

47. Puberty:

A. Peak growth velocity in girls is at breast development stage 2 to 3

B. Peak growth velocity in boys is at the 10 to 12 ml testes stage

C. Precocious puberty is usually benign in boys

D. Precocious puberty is commoner in girls

E. Delayed puberty is commoner in girls

48. Epilepsy:

A. 50% of childhood epilepsies are due to absences

B. Valproate is the drug of choice in generalised epilepsies

C. Infantile spasms occur commonly in less than three months of age

D. EEG in absence epilepsy shows a generalised three per second spike and wave pattern

E. 10% of children with infantile spasms will continue to have seizures

49. Epilepsy in childhood:

A. 95% of children with absences will have remission in adolescence

B. Most children with infantile spasms may have learning disabilities later

C. Juvenile myoclonic epilepsy is commoner in males

D. Juvenile myoclonic epilepsy usually presents between 5 to 10 years of age

E. Benign rolandic epilepsy is rare in childhood

50. Febrile convulsions:

A. Occur in 3% of children between six months and five years

B. Recurrence risk is higher in older children

C. Absolute risk of non-febrile seizure after one febrile convulsion is about 10%

D. Is associated with temporal lobe epilepsy in later childhood or adolescence

E. 50% have relatives with a seizure disorder

51. Antiepileptic drugs:

A. Sodium valproate may cause weight loss

B. Sodium valproate may cause alopecia

C. Carbamazepine may cause a lupus- like syndrome

D. Carbamazepine may cause ataxia

E. Vigabatrin may cause restriction in peripheral visual fields

52. Achondroplasia:

A. New mutations may be seen in 80% of cases

B. Is associated with deafness

C. Trident hand may be present

D. There may be associated hydrocephalus

E. Is the most common skeletal dysplasia

53. Cornelia de-Lange syndrome is associated with:

A. Tall stature

B. Generalised hirsutism

C. Undescended testes

D. Hydrocephalus

E. Limb malformation is seen in 5-10% of cases

54. Ewing's sarcoma:

A. Commonly presents as infection

B. Metastasis occurs late

C. X-ray shows periosteal elevation

D. 5 year survival is 80%

E. Surgical intervention is curative in most cases

55. Angelman syndrome:

A. Absence of paternal contribution to chromosome 15

B. There is usually mild mental retardation

C. There may be growth retardation

D. Hypotonia is a feature

E. Is associated with optic atrophy

56. Fragile- X syndrome:

A. Small head is a feature

B. Pale blue irides

C. Cryptorchidism is seen

D. Fragile site is located on the short arm of chromosome X

E. Joint laxity

57. Kallmann's syndrome (hypogonadotrophic hypogonadism):

A. Obesity is a feature

B. Hyperosmia

C. Associated with congenital renal anomalies

D. Increased risk of testicular tumours

E. Maybe X- linked recessive

58. Kallmann's syndrome:

A. Is associated with choanal atresia

B. Serum testosterone is normal

C. There may be cleft palate

D. Deafness is commonly present

E. There is no treatment

59. Congenital heart disease:

A. Ventricular septal defect is the commonest heart defect seen in Down's syndrome

B. Noonan syndrome is associated with hypertrophic obstructive cardiomyopathy

C. Pulmonary stenosis is the commonest heart defect seen in William's syndrome

D. 30% are associated with major chromosomal abnormalities

E. The overall infant cardiac surgical mortality has been reduced to 15%

60. Tetralogy of Fallot:

A. Most cases are diagnosed in the first few days of life

B. Surgical repair should be carried out as soon as possible

C. Is associated with Goldenhar syndrome (oculo-auricular-vertebral anomaly)

D. May lead to cerebral thrombosis

E. Is associated with Down's syndrome

Multiple Choice Questions- Paper 2

Decide whether each statement (A-E) is true or false.

1. Transposition of the Great Arteries (TGA):

A. The electrocardiogram is usually normal

B. A PO2 of 1 to 3 KPa is not unusual in TGA

C. TGA usually presents in the second month of life

D. Chest x-ray classically shows a boot-shaped heart

E. Surgical correction is performed at about nine months of age

2. Complications of anorexia include:

A. Renal failure

B. Parotitis

C. Carotinaemia

D. Increased bone density

E. Arrhythmias

3. Prolonged QT syndrome:

A. Is characterised by abnormal ventricular repolarisation

B. Is associated with a risk of sudden death

C. Genetic testing for it is available

D. May be misdiagnosed as epilepsy

E. May be accompanied by deafness

4. The differential diagnosis of physical abuse includes:

A. Copper deficiency

B. Impetigo

C. Ricketts

D. Osteogenesis imperfecta

E. Osteomyelitis

5. Innocent murmurs:

A. Maybe systolic or diastolic

B. Still's murmur may be confused with a VSD murmur

C. Venous hum is heard above and below the clavicles

D. Pulmonary flow murmur may be heard throughout childhood

E. Venous hum may be confused with patent ductus arteriosus

6. Congenital heart disease:

A. Maternal insulin dependent diabetes may lead to transposition of the great arteries and Truncus Arteriosus

B. Noonan syndrome is associated with hypertrophic obstructive cardiomyopathy

C. Antenatal rubella infection is associated with patent ductus arteriosus

D. Incidence is 20 per 1000 live births

E. Children with Di George's syndrome should have all vaccinations

7. Regarding the ECG in congenital heart disease:

A. In the normal neonatal ECG, there are dominant R waves in V1, and deep S waves in V6

B. Persisting neonatal RS progression after the first month implies right ventricular hypertrophy

C. A long PR interval is seen in Pompe's disease

D. A long QT is seen in hypocalcaemia

E. Prolonged PR interval is seen in hypothyroidism

8. Complications of whooping cough include:

A. Convulsions

B. Pneumonia

C. Epistaxis

D. Encephalopathy

E. Subconjunctival haemorrhage

9. Associated features of Friedreich's ataxia include:

A. Muscle tone is usually increased

B. Optic atrophy

C. Sensorineural hearing loss

D. Hypertrophic cardiomyopathy in over 60%

E. Dysarthria

10. Nitric oxide:

A. Causes vasoconstriction

B. Half-life is 3 to 6 seconds

C. Is inactivated by haemoglobin

D. Is a platelet aggregation inhibitor

E. When inhaled is useful in post-operative congenital heart disease

11. Eisenmenger's syndrome:

A. Is usually seen with atrial septal defects

B. There is a loud P2

C. Children with tetralogy of Fallot are particularly at risk

D. Patients with pulmonary atresia are protected

E. Cardiac catheterisation reveals reduced pulmonary vascular resistance

12. Patent ductus arteriosus:

A. In preterm babies there may be a systolic murmur at the left sternal border

B. May cause failure to thrive

C. If asymptomatic in the young child does not need treatment

D. There may be increased ventilatory requirement

E. Oligaemic lung fields are seen on chest x-ray

13. Marfan's syndrome is associated with:

A. Downwards subluxation of the lens

B. Strabismus

C. Pneumothorax

D. Cryptorchidism

E. Chest wall deformities

14. Causes of systemic hypertension in children include:

A. Neuroblastoma

B. Adrenogenital syndrome

C. Hypercalcaemia

D. ACTH administration

E. Mercury poisoning

15. In William's syndrome there is:

A. Autosomal dominant inheritance

B. Renal artery stenosis and hypertension

C. Tall stature

D. Stellate iris pattern

E. Normal intelligence usually

16. William's syndrome is associated with:

A. Hyperacusis

B. Neonatal hypocalcaemia

C. Enamel hypoplasia

D. Depressed nasal bridge

E. Aortic stenosis

17. Childhood psoriasis:

A. Guttate psoriasis often follows a streptococcal or viral sore throat infection

B. Fine pitting of the nails is seen commonly

C. Napkin psoriasis is a common feature of infantile psoriasis

D. Maybe familial

E. May demonstrate Von Spitz sign

18. Pityriasis rosea:

A. Viral origin

B. Begins with a single scaly macule

C. Maybe itchy

D. May follow the lines of the ribs posteriorly

E. Resolves in 4 to 6 days

19. Epidermolysis bullosa:

A. Autosomal dominant type tends to be more severe and even fatal

B. Blisters may erupt following minor trauma

C. May lead to oesophageal stenosis

D. Fingers and toes may become fused

E. Limb contractures may develop

20. Erythrasma:

A. Is caused by Corynebacterium

B. Is often seen on extensor surfaces

C. Frequently misdiagnosed as a fungal infection

D. The rash shows a coral pink fluorescence under Woods light

E. Treatment is usually not effective

21. Koebner phenomenon is seen in:

A. Lichen planus

B. Molluscum contagiosum

C. Vitiligo

D. Viral warts

E. Eczema

22. Causes of erythema multiforme:

A. Herpes simplex infection

B. Mycoplasma pneumoniae

C. HIV

D. Ebstein Barr virus

E. Lymphoma

23. Hereditary Angioedema:

A. Autosomal recessive

B. Caused by a deficiency of C1 esterase inhibitor

C. There is no urticaria

D. Is accompanied by abdominal pain

E. Usually triggered by trauma

24. Infantile seborrhoeic dermatitis:

A. Is a fungal infection

B. Rare in the first two months of life

C. Itchy

D. Child is irritable

E. Topical salicylic acid may help

25. Neonatal haemangiomas:

A. Capillary haemangiomas may be associated with glaucoma

B. Capillary haemangiomas may be associated with Klippel-Trenauney- Weber Syndrome

C. Cavernous haemangiomas grow for the first few months and then resolve

D. The strawberry naevus is associated with high output cardiac failure

E. Cavernous haemangiomas are associated with the Sturge -Webber syndrome

26. Sturge- Weber syndrome:

A. The ophthalmic division of the trigeminal nerve is always involved

B. Is associated with learning disability

C. May present with intractable epilepsy in early infancy

D. May present with hemiplegia

E. Is associated with cavernous haemangioma

27. Clinical features of mucopolysaccharidosis include:

A. Glaucoma

B. Normal development

C. Thoracic kyphosis

D. Conductive deafness

E. Valvular lesions in the heart

28. In Mucopolysaccharidosis:

A. The head is small

B. Development is usually normal up to 6 to 12 months of age

C. There is excretion of amino acids in the urine

D. Treatment with bone marrow transplant may reverse any neurological development

E. Is associated with umbilical and inguinal hernias

29. Causes of hair loss include:

A. Homocystinuria

B. Hyperthyroidism

C. Heparin therapy

D. Retinoids

E. Topical steroids

30. Rashes of infancy:

A. In candida infection of the nappy area, the flexures are characteristically spared

B. Irritant dermatitis does not occur if the napkin area is cleaned regularly

C. Irritant dermatitis may have a scalded skin appearance

D. Pityriasis rosea is not itchy

E. Acrodermatitis enteropathica causes an asymmetrical erythematous rash mainly around the mouth and anus

31. Down's syndrome:

A. Incidence is one in 5,000

B. Duodenal atresia is seen in 5 to 15%

C. 2% have Hirschsprung's disease

D. Hearing loss may be present in 10%

E. One in 1500 may have leukaemia

32. Accidental poisoning in children:

A. Occurs most commonly in children over five years of age

B. There has been a marked reduction in the hospital admission rates for accidental poisoning

C. Gastric lavage is only considered when a large quantity of a toxic drug has been taken in the previous hour

D. Activated charcoal is effective for iron, hydrocarbons and insecticides

E. Lead poisoning is the commonest cause of chronic poisoning in children

33. Lead poisoning:

A. Children may present with failure to thrive

B. it may present with seizures

C. Chronic exposure to low levels may lead to mental retardation

D. There may be polycythaemia

E. X-rays of the knee or wrist may show dense metaphyseal bands

34. Prolonged jaundice in the newborn:

A. Phototherapy is indicated in conjugated hyperbilirubinaemia

B. Hypothyroidism causes unconjugated hyperbilirubinaemia

C. Surgery for biliary atresia should be performed at six months

D. CMV and herpes cause conjugated hyperbilirubinaemia

E. Cystic fibrosis is a cause of unconjugated hyperbilirubinaemia

35. Coeliac disease:

A. Diagnosis is made on serological tests

B. May be associated with Ig G deficiency

C. Glossitis is seen

D. Siblings and offspring have a 40% risk of developing coeliac disease

E. Is associated with HLA A1 and DR3 haplotypes

36. Wilson's disease:

A. Neurological abnormalities are common in childhood

B. May be associated with Ricketts

C. Plasma caeruloplasmin is raised

D. Gene is located on chromosome 13

E. Anaemia is a feature

37. Alpha-1 antitrypsin deficiency:

A. Pulmonary disease is significant in childhood

B. Most babies present with prolonged jaundice

C. There may be intracranial haemorrhage

D. Approximately 70% of children will recover

E. Can be diagnosed antenatally

38. Alagilles's syndrome:

A. Is autosomal recessive

B. There is characteristic triangular facies

C. Aortic stenosis

D. May present with prolonged jaundice

E. Renal tubular defects

39. Viral hepatitis:

A. Interferon treatment for chronic hepatitis B is successful in 50% of children infected horizontally

B. Hepatitis B virus is an RNA virus

C. Vertical transmission of hepatitis C is rare

D. 5 to 10% of children with hepatitis C develop chronic liver disease

E. Cirrhosis develops in 50 to 70% of those with chronic hepatitis D virus infection

40. Autoimmune hepatitis:

A. More common in boys

B. Mean age of presentation is 12 to 15 years

C. Diagnosis is based on raised Ig G

D. Up to 40% of children respond to steroids and Azathioprine

E. Serum complement C4 is usually low

41. Surfactant production is:

A. Stimulated by steroids

B. Stimulated by prolactin

C. Inhibited by insulin

D. Inhibited by thyroxine

E. Inhibited by beta agonists

42. Effects of surfactant administration:

A. Causes a reduction in mortality

B. Reduces bronchopulmonary dysplasia

C. Does not affect the incidence of intraventricular haemorrhage

D. Reduces the incidence of pneumothorax

E. Reduces the incidence of pulmonary haemorrhage

43. Patent ductus arteriosus in a preterm baby:

A. Is most commonly seen with respiratory distress syndrome

B. May cause apnoea and bradycardia

C. Oxygen saturations are usually normal

D. Pulse is collapsing

E. May need fluid restriction

44. Intracranial lesions in the preterm infant:

A. Most haemorrhages occur in the first 72 hours

B. Pneumothorax is a significant risk factor for periventricular haemorrhage

C. Periventricular leukomalacia is associated with a poor outcome

D. With a normal ultrasound scan, there is a 25% chance of being normal

E. The majority of periventricular haemorrhages are harmless

45. Necrotising enteropathic colitis:

A. Feeding should be with milk only

B. There may be bile- stained vomiting

C. Ventilatory support may be required

D. Characteristic features on x-ray are thin- walled bowel loops with perforations

E. Mortality is 75%

46. Problems relating to prematurity:

A. Retinopathy of prematurity is first detected at the equivalent of 26 weeks gestational age

B. Retinopathy of prematurity occurs in 20% of all very low birth weight infants

C. Severe visual impairment occurs in about 15% of very low birth weight babies

D. Chronic lung disease of prematurity is defined as additional oxygen requirement beyond 36 weeks gestational age

E. Chest x-ray in chronic lung disease charity characteristically shows fibrosis and cystic changes

47. Kernicterus:

A. Is caused by the deposition of conjugated bilirubin in the basal ganglia

B. The baby may lie in opisthotonus position

C. May lead to choreoathetoid cerebral palsy

D. Paralysis of upward gaze

E. May cause discolouration of the teeth which improves

48. Diaphragmatic hernia:

A. Occurs in about one in 10,000 births

B. Usually presents as respiratory distress with failure to respond to resuscitation

C. Is associated with pneumothorax

D. Lung hyperplasia is the main cause of the high mortality

E. Has a mortality rate of 10 %

49. Neonatal sepsis may present with:

A. Hypothermia

B. Hyperglycaemia

C. Neutropenia

D. Opisthotonus posture

E. Meconium staining of the liquor at birth

50. Cleft lip and palate:

A. Incidence is 10 per 1000 babies

B. Surgical repair of the palate is carried out within the first week of life

C. Infants are prone to acute otitis media

D. Adenoidectomy may be indicated

E. Can be detected antenatally

51. Pierre- Robin sequence:

A. Is associated with cleft palate

B. Is associated with congenital heart disease

C. Autosomal recessive

D. May result in cyanotic episodes

E. Prone-positioning helps

52. Exomphalos and Gastroschisis:

A. Gastroschisis is commonly associated with other congenital abnormalities

B. Gastroschisis is more common in females

C. In exomphalos the bowel protrudes through a defect in the anterior abdominal wall adjacent to the umbilicus

D. in Gastroschisis, the bowel is covered with peritoneum

E. Exomphalos is associated with Turner's syndrome

53. Congenital gastrointestinal disorders:

A. 8% of oesophageal atresias occur with a tracheo-oesophageal fistula

B. Oesophageal atresia presents with persistent salivation

C. A child with Hirschsprung's disease may present as an acute enterocolitis

D. In small bowel obstruction there is persistent vomiting which is bile stained if the obstruction is above the ampulla of Vater

E. Are seen in Beckwith-Wiedemann Syndrome

54. Beckwith-Wiedemann Syndrome is associated with:

A. Autosomal dominant inheritance

B. Increased incidence of Wilm's tumour

C. Neonatal hyperglycaemia

D. Omphalocoele

E. Microcephaly

55. Childhood malignancies:

A. Lymphomas are the commonest malignancy in childhood

B. Retinoblastoma is associated with a deletion on chromosome 13

C. Childhood cancer is commoner in boys

D. Neuroblastoma and Wilm's tumour usually present at 5 to 10 years of age

E. Cancer is the second commonest cause of deaths in children

56. Acute lymphoblastic leukaemia:

A. Accounts for 50% of leukaemia in children

B. The blood count is always abnormal

C. Age more than 10 years is associated with good prognosis

D. Philadelphia chromosome is associated with better prognosis

E. Chemotherapy is continued for up to 3 years

57. Lymphoma:

A. Hodgkin's disease is more common in childhood than non- Hodgkin's lymphoma

B. B-cell non-Hodgkin's lymphoma typically present as a mediastinal mass

C. Reed-Sternberg cells are pathognomonic of non-Hodgkin's lymphoma

D. Hodgkin's disease usually presents with enlarged lymph nodes in the neck

E. Previous exposure to the Epstein-Barr virus is a risk factor for Hodgkin's disease

58. Neuroblastoma:

A. Spontaneous regression may occur in very young infants

B. Most common between 5 to 10 years of age

C. May present with spinal cord compression

D. Most children over one year have poor prognosis

E. Expression of the N-myc oncogene is associated with better prognosis

59. Wilm's tumour:

A. Is associated with aniridia

B. Is commonly seen after 10 years of age

C. The child is usually well

D. Commonly presents with haematuria and hypertension

E. The overall prognosis is 50% of patients are cured

60. Nephrotic syndrome:

A. Is more common in girls

B. 85% are due to minimal change disease

C. May occur secondary to malaria

D. Is often precipitated by respiratory infections

E. Membranous nephropathy is associated with hepatitis B

Multiple Choice Questions- Paper 3

Decide whether each statement (A-E) is true or false.

1. Bone tumours in childhood:

A. Ewing's sarcoma is seen more often in younger children
B. Malignant bone tumours are commonly seen up to 12 years of age
C. The limbs are the most common site
D. Most patients are well
E. Are difficult to treat

2. Retinoblastoma:

A. Most present within the first three years of life
B. Is associated with mutations on chromosome 13
C. Maybe familial
D. Leukocoria is seen in 90%
E. There is a significant risk of second malignancy

3. Prune- belly syndrome:

A. Is commoner in females

B. Associated with congenital dislocation of the hips

C. Associated with chromosomal defect on number 11

D. May be associated with cryptorchidism

E. Pulmonary hyperplasia is a feature.

4. Urinary tract infection:

A. Proteus infection is more common in girls

B. Proteus infection predisposes to the formation of phosphate stones

C. Pseudomonas infection is an indicator of structural abnormality in the urinary tract

D. UTI in infancy may present with prolonged neonatal jaundice

E. Vesicoureteric reflux is familial

5. Henoch-Schonlein Purpura:

A. Is often preceded by an upper respiratory infection

B. The rash is characteristically palpable

C. Orchitis is a known complication

D. Intussusception may occur

E. Follow up is necessary

6. Horner's syndrome:

A. There is anhidrosis of the contralateral side of the face

B. Exophthalmos is a feature
C. Heterochromia of the iris is seen
D. May be caused by a Neuroblastoma
E. May be caused by brachial plexus damage at birth

7. Tall stature may be caused by:

A. Obesity

B. Congenital adrenal hyperplasia

C. Homocysteinuria

D. Soto's syndrome

E. Beckwith- Wiedemann syndrome

8. Cerebral palsy:

A. Is a progressive lesion of the motor pathways

B. Is the commonest cause of motor impairment in children

C. Learning difficulties are present in 90%

D. Epilepsy is present in 40%

E. Visual impairment is seen in 50%

9. In whooping cough:

A. Whoop often presents in infants

B. Apnoea may follow paroxysms in babies

C. Vomiting may be a feature

D. Erythromycin may be used for prophylaxis

E. Salbutamol, steroids and anti-tussives have no proven role

10. Cerebral palsy:

A. In ataxic hypotonic cerebral palsy, there are asymmetric in- coordinate movements

B. Ataxic hypotonic cerebral palsy is commonly due to a genetic cause

C. There is moderate to severe intellectual impairment in dyskinetic cerebral palsy

D. Abnormal movements are seen in early infancy and dyskinetic cerebral palsy

E. In the dyskinetic type there is damage to the basal ganglia

11. Ataxia telangiectasia:

A. Is autosomal dominant

B. Telangiectasia is present from five years of age

C. There is raised serum alpha- fetoprotein

D. Is associated with hypergammaglobulinaemia

E. Failure to thrive is seen

12. Friedreich's ataxia:

A. Is autosomal dominant

B. Presents with progressive clumsiness

C. There is proximal muscle weakness

D. Impairment of joint position and vibration sense

E. Is associated with diabetes mellitus

13. Causes of a long PR interval include:

A. Duchenne's muscular dystrophy

B. High fever

C. Myotonic dystrophy

D. Ebstein's anomaly

E. Diphtheria

14. Cerebral haemorrhage:

A. Extradural haemorrhage is usually associated with a skull fracture

B. In young children, initial presentation of an extradural haemorrhage may be with anaemia and shock.

C. Subarachnoid haemorrhage may present with a fever

D. Lumbar puncture should be done in subarachnoid haemorrhage

E. Subdural haematoma is seen almost exclusively in non-accidental injuries in infants

15. Contra-indications to breastfeeding include:

A. Mastitis

B. Hepatitis B

C. Tuberculosis on treatment

D. Baby with galactosaemia

E. Lithium treatment

16. Long-term management of diabetes in children includes:

A. Annual blood pressure checks from diagnosis if aged five years onwards

B. Microalbuminuria annually from 18 years

C. Annual retinopathy from 12 years

D. The target HbA1C is less than 7.5%

E. Screening for coeliac disease should be done every three years

17. Guillain-Barre syndrome (acute post –infectious polyneuropathy) :

    A. Peak age in childhood is 4 to 7 years

    B. May occur after Campylobacter gastroenteritis

    C. There is autonomic involvement

    D. The CSF white cell count is raised

    E. Cranial nerves may be involved

18. In Guillain-Barre syndrome:

A. There is ascending asymmetrical weakness

B. Reflexes may be absent

C. Loss of proprioception and vibratory sensation precedes loss of pain and touch

D. Steroids have been shown to have a beneficial effect

E. 90% recover within six months

19. Bell's palsy:

A. Is usually post viral infection

B. Is associated with coarctation of the aorta

C. In an upper motor neuron lesion, the child cannot wrinkle their forehead

D. There is strong evidence for the use of steroids

E. The main complication is conjunctivitis

20. Juvenile myasthenia:

A. Is of autoimmune aetiology

B. May present with ophthalmoplegia

C. Usually presents before 10 years of age

D. Weakness improves with exercise

E. Azathioprine has been shown to be of value

21. Neurofibromatosis:

A. Up to 50% are due to new mutations

B. Neurofibromata may involve the cranial nerves

C. Type I is associated with mental retardation

D. Type I is coded on chromosome 22

E. Is associated with renal artery stenosis

22. Tuberous sclerosis:

A. Is associated with cardiac rhabdomyomata

B. Café au lait patches are present in 25% of cases

C. There may be gingival fibromas

D. Subungual fibromas are commonly seen in childhood

E. Mental retardation is seen in 20%

23. Mucopolysaccharidosis:

A. Is associated with developmental regression

B. There may be glaucoma

C. Claw hand may be seen

D. Is associated with sensorineural deafness

E. May lead to cardiac failure

24. In Dermatomyositis:

A. Anterior neck flexures and trunk muscles are typically involved

B. Post-exercise pain is seen rarely

C. Rash may be seen on the flexor surfaces of joints

D. There is acute onset of progressive muscle weakness

E. ESR is usually normal

25. Myotonic dystrophy:

A. Is autosomal recessive

B. Mental development is normal

C. Cardiomyopathy may co-exist

D. Is associated with diabetes mellitus

E. Presents with hypertonia at birth

26. Infectious mononucleosis:

A. Splenomegaly is seen in up to 20%

B. Maculopapular rash is a feature in 10% if given ampicillin

C. Jaundice may be a feature

D. Diagnosis is supported by the presence of heterophil antibodies

E. Symptoms may persist for one to 3 months

27. Human herpes virus:

A. Primary human herpes virus 8 is a common cause of febrile convulsions

B. Roseola infantum is caused by human herpes virus 8

C. Aseptic meningitis is usually due to herpes simplex virus 2 infections

D. Encephalitis due to herpes simplex virus usually resolves without sequelae

E. Herpes simplex virus involving the eye may lead to loss of vision

28. Mumps:

A. Is spread by saliva

B. Incubation period is 7 to 14 days

C. Plasma amylase is often elevated

D. May lead to permanent hearing loss

E. Orchitis is a common complication in pre-pubertal males

29. The following viruses are droplet- spread:

A. Epstein Barr virus

B. Varicella

C. Pox virus

D. Human papilloma virus

E. Coxsackie virus

30. Macrocephaly is seen in:

A. Inborn errors of metabolism

B. Trisomy 21

C. Soto's syndrome

D. Mucopolysaccharidosis

E. Postnatal encephalitis

31. Meningitis:

A. Meningococcal infection has the highest risk of long-term neurological sequelae

B. Pneumococcal meningitis is associated with a low risk of morbidity and mortality

C. Meningitis is minimal in tuberculous meningitis

D. Tuberculous meningitis is associated with a high mortality and morbidity

E. Rifampicin is given as prophylaxis against meningococcal meningitis to all school and work colleagues.

32. Childhood tics:

A. Are entirely involuntary

B. Worsen when the child is actively concentrating

C. There is often a family history

D. May require medication

E. May be an emotional reaction

33. Diabetes in children:

A. Is diagnosed with a fasting glucose

B. Affects around 10 per 1000 children by 16 years of age

C. Mono neuropathy may involve the cranial nerves

D. Is associated with Prader- Willi syndrome

E. The peak age at presentation is 6-8 years

34. Inborn errors of metabolism:

A. May present in the neonatal period with persistent vomiting

B. Phenylketonuria may present with infantile spasms

C. Homocysteinuria may present with upwards subluxation of the ocular lens

D. There may be pendular nystagmus in albinism

E. Galactosaemia may present with hyperglycaemia

35. Sickle cell disease:

A. Is associated with delayed puberty

B. Is associated with sleep apnoea syndrome

C. Pneumococcal vaccine should be given at one year of age

D. Vaso- occlusive crises will be prevented if the proportion of HbS is 50%

E. Exchange transfusion is indicated for priapism

36. Complications of obesity include:

A. Slipped upper femoral epiphysis

B. Sleep apnoea

C. Benign intracranial hypertension

D. Heart failure

E. Diabetes mellitus

37. Regarding growth in children:

A. The fetal phase of growth accounts for about 30% of eventual height

B. Extreme intra-uterine growth retardation can result in permanent short stature

C. Chronic unhappiness may result in short stature

D. Obesity may lead to poor stature

E. Normal growth velocity of children over 2 years is 5cm/ year.

38. Normal puberty:

A. The first sign in girls is the onset of menstruation

B. The first sign in boys is deepening in voice and growth of facial hair

C. The height spurt in boys occurs when the testicular volume reaches 4 ml

D. Bone age measurement is usually done from an x-ray of the humerus or femur

E. Puberty ceases with epiphyseal closure

39. Causes of precocious puberty include:

A. Hydrocephalus

B. Hyperthyroidism

C. Leydig cell tumour of the testis

D. Neurofibromatosis

E. Craniopharyngioma

40. Congenital adrenal hyperplasia:

A. There is a raised level of 21 hydroxylase in the blood

B. Leads to tall stature in males

C. Is associated with metabolic alkalosis

D. Hypoglycaemia occurs in a salt- losing crisis

E. Prenatal diagnosis is possible

41. Irritable hip:

A. Is the most common cause of acute hip pain in children

B. Often follows a viral infection

C. There is pain at rest

D. There may be a mild fever

E. May be associated with pain in the knee

42. Features of Osteogenesis imperfecta include:

A. Autosomal dominant inheritance

B. Blue sclera

C. Hearing loss

D. Fractures may be present before birth

E. Type II is associated with a poor prognosis

43. Perthe's disease:

A. Occurs most commonly at 10 to 15 years of age

B. Is more common in girls

C. Magnetic resonance imaging may be required for diagnosis

D. Prognosis is generally poor

E. Treatment is usually surgical

44. Slipped upper femoral epiphysis:

A. Is seen in tall thin children

B. Most common at 5 to 10 years of age

C. The leg is shortened and externally rotated

D. Is unilateral in 25%

E. Treatment is with bed rest and splints

45. Slipped upper femoral epiphysis may occur in association with:

A. Hyperthyroidism

B. Pseudo-hypopituitarism

C. Obesity

D. Delayed puberty

E. Growth hormone disorders

46. Talipes equinovarus:

A. The birth prevalence is 10 per 1000 live births

B. Is associated with developmental dysplasia of the hip

C. Is commoner in females

D. Corrective surgery is performed at 6 to 9 weeks of age

E. May be associated with spina bifida

47. The following conditions are autosomal dominant:

A. Wilson's disease

B. Infantile polycystic renal failure

C. Peutz-Jegher's disease

D. Adult polycystic kidney disease

E. Hereditary spherocytosis

48. Regarding congenital infections:

A. Cytomegalovirus can cause cataracts

B. Toxoplasma may cause congenital heart defects

C. Cytomegalovirus may cause sensorineural deafness

D. Toxoplasma causes retinopathy which may lead to blindness

E. Babies born to mothers who develop chickenpox within five days of delivery need Zoster immunoglobulin and acyclovir

49. Regarding developmental milestones:

A. Transfers at 3 months

B. Mouthing at 9 months

C. Pincer grip at 12 months

D. Builds a tower of 8 bricks at 15 months

E. Copies a triangle at 3 years

50. The following are autosomal recessive:

A. Protein C deficiency

B. Von Willebrand disease

C. Gilbert's disease

D. Hyperlipidaemia

E. Alpha1- antitrypsin deficiency

51. The following are X linked recessive diseases:

A. Duchenne muscular dystrophy

B. Myotonic dystrophy

C. Galactosaemia

D. Glucose 6 phosphate dehydrogenase deficiency

E. Haemochromatosis

52. Human Papilloma virus (HPV) vaccination:

A. Cevarix protects against genital warts as well as cervical cancer

B. Efficacy is more than 99%

C. Gardasil is licensed from nine years

D. If the course is interrupted it should be repeated

E. Is contra- indicated in HIV infection

53. Sudden infant death syndrome:

A. Incidence has increased

B. Occurs most commonly at 4 to 6 months of age

C. 60% are normal birth weight term infants

D. 80% of affected mothers are more than 20 years old

E. Is associated with high maternal parity

54. The child's social environment (in the UK):

A. About 15% of Afro-Caribbean children live in a single-parent household

B. The under 18 conception rate in the UK is 10 per 1000

C. Over 40% of 15-year-olds consume alcohol

D. 15% of 15-year-olds have had personal experience of using drugs

E. 30% of children smoke regularly

55. The following are DNA viruses:

A. Parvovirus B 19

B. Rotavirus

C. Hepatitis C virus

D. Cytomegalovirus

E. Epstein-Barr virus

56. Atrial septal defect:

A. May present with recurrent chest infections

B. Arrhythmias are common in the first decade

C. May be a feature in fetal alcohol syndrome

D. Is associated with oligaemic lung fields on chest x-ray

E. There is right axis deviation on ECG

57. Ventricular septal defects:

A. Muscular type is commoner

B. Large defects are associated with loud pan-systolic murmurs

C. Heart failure usually presents at six months of age

D. Large defects always lead to pulmonary hypertension

E. Pulmonary hypertension may be evident as upright T waves on ECG

58. Pulmonary stenosis:

A. Most children are symptomatic

B. May be caused by maternal ingestion of Phenytoin antenatally

C. Is associated with Noonan syndrome

D. Is seen in congenital rubella

E. May be a feature in neurofibromatosis

59. Aortic stenosis:

A. Most are asymptomatic

B. Pulse is low-volume

C. Children usually have failure to thrive

D. Is a feature of William's syndrome

E. Is commoner in girls

60. Tetralogy of Fallot:

A. May present with inconsolable crying

B. May be seen in fetal alcohol syndrome

C. Chest x-ray classically shows a boot- shaped heart

D. May lead to Eisenmenger's syndrome

E. There is a left-to-right shunt

Multiple Choice Questions- Paper 4

Decide whether each statement (A-E) is true or false.

1. **Tetralogy of Fallot:**

   A. Often presents with heart failure
   B. Ejection systolic murmur is most prominent during a Tet spell
   C. Cerebral vascular accidents may occur in children with tetralogy of Fallot, less than two years old
   D. Cerebral abscess is a known complication
   E. Is associated with anaemia

2. **Some important "limit ages":**

   A. Not reaching for objects at four months
   B. Not walking unaided at 18 months
   C. Not saying single words with meaning at 15 months
   D. No 2 to 3 word sentences at 24 months
   E. Not achieved good eye contact at three months

3. **Sleep apnoea:**

   A. May lead to pulmonary hypertension
   B. May lead to failure to thrive
   C. May lead to developmental delay
   D. May lead to daytime somnolence

E. Adeno- tonsillectomy rarely helps

4. Cystic fibrosis:

A. The gene is located on chromosome 9

B. Diabetes is common in the first 5 years

C. A high-fat diet is recommended

D. May present with prolonged jaundice in infancy

E. Is associated with nasal polyps

5. Asthma:

A. Affects 5% of school children in the UK

B. In childhood is commoner in females

C. Causes 15 to 20 deaths in children per year in the UK

D. The main symptom in the preschool child is nocturnal cough

E. Most children over five years can use a peak flow meter

6. Acute abdominal pain in children:

A. Intussusception may lead to hypovolaemic shock

B. The success rate of reducing an intussusception by rectal air insufflation is about 25%

C. Meckel's diverticulum may present with severe rectal bleeding

D. Mesenteric adenitis is a common cause

E. Malrotation may present with dark green vomiting in the first few days of life

7. Recurrent abdominal pain:

A. An organic cause can be found in 25%

B. The pain is characteristically around the umbilicus

C. Investigations are usually abnormal

D. Pizotifen is a helpful prophylactic agent in abdominal migraine

E. In 25% the symptoms persist till adulthood

8. Coeliac disease:

A. A positive IgA gliadin titre is very specific for coeliac disease

B. IgA tissue transglutaminase has a sensitivity of 95% for Coeliac disease

C. There is increased risk in patients with IgM deficiency

D. The increased risk of intestinal lymphoma in adulthood is reduced to normal by adhering to a gluten-free diet

E. The frequency is increasing in the UK

9. Causes of raised sweat sodium include:

A. Hyperthyroidism

B. Glucose 6 phosphate dehydrogenase deficiency

C. Nephrotic syndrome

D. Severe malnutrition

E. Diabetes mellitus

10. Lyme disease:

A. Manifests as erythema migrans

B. May lead to cranial nerve palsies

C. Joint disease occurs in about 10%

D. May lead to heart block

E. The drug of choice in children over 12 years is doxycycline

11. Kawasaki's disease:

A. Peak ages 2 to 3 years

B. Is much more common in Caucasians

C. Older children are more severely affected

D. Is caused by a bacteria

E. Is a form of vasculitis

12. Examples of secondary prevention are:

A. Cycling helmets

B. Guthrie test

C. Teaching parents first aid skills

D. Speed limits

E. Blister packs for prescription medicines

13. Examples of primary prevention are:

A. Teaching road safety

B. Seat belts

C. Child resistant lids

D. Immunisations

E. Smoke alarms

14. Sickle cell disease:

A. Presents at birth

B. The child is usually very unwell due to symptoms from anaemia

C. Is the most common cause of stroke in children

D. Need prophylaxis with penicillin

E. Pneumococcal vaccination is recommended

15. Pyloric stenosis:

A. Is more common in firstborns

B. Hyperkalaemia may be present

C. There is metabolic acidosis

D. The incidence is one in 150 males

E. Indirect hyperbilirubinaemia may be present

16. Kallmann's syndrome is associated with:

A. Delayed puberty

B. Mental retardation

C. No response to gonadotropin releasing hormone stimulation

D. Cleft lip

E. Chromosome pattern is 47 XXY

17. Causes of a prolonged QT on ECG are:

A. Myocarditis

B. Hypercalcaemia

C. Head injury

D. High fever

E. Erythromycin

18. Jaundice in the newborn:

A. Toxoplasmosis causes conjugated hyperbilirubinaemia

B. Alpha-1 antitrypsin deficiency is a cause of unconjugated hyperbilirubinaemia

C. May be seen in 30 to 40% of normal term neonates

D. Is commoner in exclusively breastfed babies

E. Phototherapy is used to treat conjugated hyperbilirubinaemia

19. Primitive reflexes:

A. Moro reflex disappears at three months

B. Red reflex indicates the presence of Retinoblastoma

C. Rooting reflex persists up to nine months

D. Grasping reflex persists to six months

E. Stepping reflex persists to six months

20. Sudden infant death syndrome:

A. Incidence is five per 1000 live births

B. Minor infection is a risk factor

C. Females are at higher risk

D. Using a pacifier may be protective

E. If the baby was a twin the surviving twin should be investigated

21. Chickenpox:

A. An infected child should be excluded from school till the rash disappears

B. Zoster immunoglobulin should be given to the baby if the mother develops chickenpox two days after delivery

C. Life-threatening pneumonitis is a recognised complication

D. Incubation period is approximately a week

E. Aciclovir should be given routinely

22. Duchenne muscular dystrophy:

A. 25% are wheelchair dependent by 12 years

B. Learning disability is rare

C. Dystrophin is seen on muscle biopsy and is used for diagnosis

D. Females are asymptomatic

E. Death is usually from respiratory failure

23. Infantile spasms:

A. Onset is in the first 12 months

B. May lead to developmental regression

C. Are more common in males

D. Electroencephalogram is usually normal

E. Characteristically presents with sudden flexion of the body

24. Generalised epilepsy:

A. Absence seizures show bursts of 3 cycles per second spike and wave activity on electroencephalogram (EEG)

B. Infantile spasms are associated with a normal EEG

C. Complex partial seizures are characterised by nocturnal partial seizures

D. Benign rolandic epilepsy is characterised by stereotypical behaviour

E. Sodium valproate is the drug of choice in absence seizures

25. Speech development:

A. A normally developing child would have a six word vocabulary by two years

B. Singing nursery rhymes by four years

C. Speech delay may be a sign of autism

D. Speech and language problems are more common in boys

E. Echolalia is normal at 15 months

26. Treatment of asthma:

A. Long acting beta agonists are added in at step three of children less than five years old

B. Leukotriene inhibitors may reduce the amount of steroid needed

C. Should start at step one and stepped up as necessary

D. Turbohaler is appropriate for use in a four year old

E. Metered dose inhaler with face mask is needed less than 2 years

27. Squints:

A. Are common, occurring in approximately 10% of children

B. Maybe a sign of retinoblastoma

C. Paralytic squint is the most common form

D. In the cover test, if the uncovered eye moves to fix on the object, it is a latent squint

E. There is strong familial incidence

28. Depression in childhood:

A. Is more common in males

B. Suicide is the third leading cause of death in adolescence

C. Deliberate self harm is commoner in females

D. May manifest as primary enuresis

E. Chronic physical disease may be a predisposing factor

29. BCG:

A. Gives approximately 50% protection

B. Is contraindicated in Di George syndrome

C. The tuberculin test may be negative in flu

D. Vaccination may result in disseminated disease

E. Should not be given to a child whose mother is pregnant

30. Clubfoot:

A. Is commoner in males

B. Can be genetically inherited

C. Serial splinting helps

D. Is associated with genu valgum or varum

E. 25% are bilateral

31. Signs of physical abuse typically include:

A. Perforated eardrum

B. Spiral fracture of the humerus

C. Torn frenulum

D. Bruises over the shins

E. Mongolian blue spot

32. Regarding faltering growth:

A. Occurs across all socio economic groups

B. Most cases have an organic cause

C. Emotional deprivation is a major reason

D. Healthy babies should be weighed twice a month up to 6 months

E. The child may need to be hospitalised to observe feeding

33. Attention deficit hyperactivity disorder:

A. Intelligence is reduced

B. There may be disturbance of communication including language and comprehension

C. Is characterised by stereotypical behaviour

D. Is more common in boys

E. Is associated with food additives

34. The following are notifiable diseases:

A. Campylobacter

B. Scarlet fever

C. Tuberculosis

D. Tetanus

E. Meningitis

35. Obesity:

A. Is associated with Prader- Willi syndrome

B. Is associated with hyperinsulinism

C. Slipped upper femoral epiphyses is a known complication

D. Can be caused by excessive growth hormone

E. Hypothalamic damage is a known cause

36. Constipation:

A. Coeliac disease may present with constipation

B. Is associated with Down's syndrome

C. Is seen in spina bifida

D. Rectal biopsy may be needed

E. Laxatives are used short-term

37. Phenylketonuria:

A. There is decreased pigmentation

B. Mentation is normal

C. Incidence is one in 1000

D. Dietary restriction is the mainstay of treatment

E. Dietary restriction is not needed during pregnancy in affected girls

38. Dentition:

A. Is delayed in Rickets

B. Hutchinson's teeth occur due to congenital rubella infection

C. Primary teeth begin to appear at three months

D. All natal teeth should be removed

E. Fever and diarrhoea is normal in teething

39. The following drugs are safe in breastfeeding:

A. Temazepam

B. Nitrofurantoin

C. Ranitidine

D. Chloramphenicol

E. Sulphasalazine

40. Primary prevention programs include:

A. The Back- to- sleep program for prevention of cot death

B. The Guthrie test

C. Reducing parental smoking

D. Breastfeeding promotion

E. Newborn hearing screen

41. Causes of tall stature include:

A. Soto's syndrome

B. Hyperthyroidism

C. Noonan's syndrome

D. Cushing's syndrome

E. Klinefelter's syndrome

42. Atopic eczema:

A. Usually presents in the first six months of life

B. Is associated with Pityriasis alba

C. 50% resolve by three years

D. Antihistamines help with itching

E. Is associated with Keratosis pilaris

43. Acute bronchiolitis:

A. The evidence for use of bronchodilators is strong

B. Is caused by respiratory syncytial virus in up to half of cases

C. Is linked to maternal smoking

D. Breastfeeding helps

E. Post bronchiolitis wheeze occurs in up to 50%

44. Cot death:

A. The use of apnoea monitors decreases the incidence of cot death

B. Using a pacifier (dummy) increases the risk

C. Prone sleeping is preventative

D. Viral illness is a risk factor

E. Highest incidence is in the first month of life

45. Autism:

A. Learning disability is an associated feature

B. Usually develops between 3 to 5 years

C. May present with speech delay

D. Majority have normal IQ (intelligence quotient)

E. Is associated with visual and hearing impairment

46. Gastro-oesophageal reflux disease:

A. Frequently presents with apnoea and bradycardia

B. is associated with cerebral palsy

C. Is caused by fast transit through the stomach

D. Is associated with a solid diet

E. May present with dystonic posture

47. Precocious puberty:

A. Is almost always pathological in boys

B. Is seen in neurofibromatosis

C. Premature thelarche is usually seen between 5 to 8 years

D. Leads to short stature

E. Gonadotropin hormone releasing hormone analogues are used to treat it

48. HIV:

A. 5% of children with HIV develop AIDS each year

B. Vertical transmission rate with no intervention is 50%

C. All children less than two years should be started on treatment regardless of the CD 4 count

D. AIDS is a notifiable disease

E. Vaginal delivery is allowed

49. Rickets:

A. Liver disease is a causative factor

B. Dentition is delayed

C. Weight- bearing milestones are delayed

D. Children have short attention span

E. Is seen in Fanconi's anaemia

50. Typical presentation of non- accidental head injury includes:

A. Extra- dural haemorrhage

B. Retinal haemorrhages

C. Feeding difficulties

D. Children aged 1 to 3 years

E. Bilateral black eyes

51. MMR vaccine:

A. Can be given to a child who had a bone marrow transplant within six months

B. Is contraindicated in egg allergy

C. Is contraindicated if allergic to neomycin

D. May lead to parotid swelling in 10%

E. Idiopathic thrombocytopenic purpura may occur within thirty days of having the vaccine

52. Cystic fibrosis:

A. The lungs are defective at birth

B. Diabetes is a known complication

C. Up to 50% of cases have nasal polyps

D. Is associated with rectal prolapse

E. Carrier frequency is 1: 50

53. Ring worm:

A. Tinea corporis causes annular lesions

B. Tinea capitis results in hair loss

C. Tinea capitis shows up as fluorescent green under Wood's light

D. Tinea pedis usually requires oral griseofulvin

E. Topical agents are effective for Tinea capitis

54. Statistics:

A. Incidence is the total number of cases in the population at any one time

B. Sensitivity is the percentage of those who do not have a condition, who are correctly tested negative

C. Positive likelihood ratio is a positive test in an affected individual compared with a positive result in an un-affected individual

D. A statistically significant result indicates high clinical significance

E. The smaller the p value, the more significant the result

55. Common viral infections:

A. Coxsackie virus A16 causes vesicles on the hands

B. In parvovirus B 19 infection, aplastic anaemia is a recognised complication

C. Glandular fever can be treated with amoxicillin

D. Mumps virus affects the B lymphocytes

E. Roseola infantum (HHV-6) accounts for a third of cases with febrile convulsions under one year of age

56. Non-gastrointestinal manifestations of coeliac disease include:

A. Hirsutism

B. Precocious puberty

C. Stomatitis

D. Neuropathy

E. Dermatitis herpetiformis

57. Acne:

A. Neonatal acne is common

B. Needs investigation if initial presentation is between 1 to 7 years

C. Girls are more commonly affected

D. Is caused by a bacterium

E. Isotretinoin can be tried before referral to secondary care

58. Consent:

A. Parental consent is needed up to 18 years

B. A Gillick competent 16-year-old may refuse treatment for life threatening disease

C. Preschool children should be involved in the process of consent

D. A 14-year-old has the right to confidentiality

E. An unmarried father cannot consent to treatment for his child

59. Hip pain:

A. Inguinal hernia may be a cause

B. Due to septic arthritis commonly presents in young children

C. Irritable hip commonly affects children aged 5 to 8 years

D. Due to Perthes disease is usually bilateral

E. Irritable hip is usually of viral aetiology

60. Breast-feeding reduces the incidence of:

A. Respiratory infections

B. Infantile colic

C. Diabetes in the infant

D. Otitis media

E. Necrotising enterocolitis in low birth weight babies

Multiple Choice Questions Paper – 5

Decide whether each statement (A-E) is true or false.

1. Rubella:

A. Characteristic sub-occipital lymphadenopathy appears after the rash

B. Infection in the first eight weeks of gestation will result in fetal death in approximately 60%

C. Hydrocephalus and calcification in the brain are characteristically seen in congenital rubella

D. Retinopathy in congenital rubella does not affect vision

E. Rash begins on the trunk and spreads to the face

2. Learning disability occurs in:

A. Duchenne muscular dystrophy

B. Angelman's syndrome

C. Turner syndrome

D. Achondroplasia

E. Marfan's syndrome

3. Homocystinuria is associated with:

A. Hyper-mobile joints

B. Upward subluxation of the lens

C. Short stature

D. Thrombosis

E. Normal IQ

4. Non-epileptic seizures:

A. Breath- holding attacks may be voluntary

B. Vomiting may precipitate a reflex anoxic seizure

C. Psychogenic seizures may lead to epileptiform attacks

D. Reflex anoxic seizures may continue as the child grows older

E. Psychogenic seizures may lead to sudden muscular jerks

5. Effects on the infant of poorly controlled diabetes in the mother include:

A. Polycythaemia

B. Sacral agenesis

C. Hypercalcaemia

D. Imperforate anus

E. Renal agenesis

6. Differential diagnosis of non-accidental fractures includes:

A. Osteogenesis imperfecta

B. Rickets

C. Vitamin A and C deficiency

D. Achondroplasia

E. Renal disease

7. Predisposing factors to abuse include:

A. Learning disability in parents

B. History of difficult pregnancy

C. Pre-maturity

D. Admission of baby to special care baby unit

E. Having extended family nearby

8. Regarding chest x-ray findings:

A. Egg-on- side cardiac outline is seen in tetralogy of Fallot

B. Oligaemic lung fields in pulmonary stenosis

C. Boot- shaped heart is seen in transposition of the great arteries

D. Cardiomegaly due to atrial septal defect

E. Plethoric lung fields in ventricular septal defect

9. Causes of a prolonged QT interval on ECG include:

A. Hyperkalaemia

B. Diphtheria

C. Congenital

D. High fever more than 40°C

E. Domperidone

10. Causes of a long PR interval include:

A. Ventricular septal defect

B. Erythromycin

C. Eisenmenger's syndrome

D. Dilated cardiomyopathy

E. Kawasaki disease

11. Rheumatic fever:

A. Incidence is increasing

B. Erythema marginatum is a major criterion for diagnosis

C. Subcutaneous nodules is a minor criteria for diagnosis

D. Needs antibiotic prophylaxis for 25 years

E. May lead to prolonged QT interval

12. Congenital heart disease:

A. 80 to 90% of small ventricular septal defects are asymptomatic

B. Coarctation of the aorta is a common diagnosis

C. Tetralogy of Fallot should be repaired within 6 to 9 weeks of life

D. In atrial septal defect the ECG shows partial right bundle branch block in 90%

E. Atrial septal defects should be closed surgically within the first year of life

13. Complications of maternal diabetes in the infant include:

A. Renal vein thrombosis

B. Hyperbilirubinaemia

C. Anaemia

D. Duodenal atresia

E. Neural tube defects

14. Toe- walking:

A. Is common up to 3 years of age

B. Is seen in Duchenne muscular dystrophy

C. Can be due to infantile autism

D. Is seen in spina bifida

E. Seen in peroneal muscle atrophy

15. Cephalhaematoma:

A. The overlying skin is bruised and oedematous

B. Disappears over a few days

C. Is present at birth

D. Is limited by suture lines

E. No treatment is needed

16. Kawasaki disease:

A. Is of viral aetiology

B. Cervical lymphadenopathy is one of the diagnostic criteria

C. Thrombocytosis occurs early

D. Coronary artery aneurysms occur in up to 40%

E. Mortality is 5%

17. Café au- lait spots are associated with:

A. Fanconi's anaemia

B. Normal variant

C. Tuberous sclerosis

D. Friedreich's ataxia

E. Russell- Silver syndrome

18. Macrocephaly may be caused by:

A. Neurofibromatosis

B. Meningitis

C. Trisomy 13

D. Anaemia

E. Galactosaemia

19. Hypotonia in the infant is seen in:

A. Spina bifida

B. Kernicterus

C. Prader- Willi syndrome

D. Birth asphyxia

E. Trisomy 18

20. Complications of insulin-dependent diabetes in children include:

A. Mood change and irritability

B. Coeliac disease

C. Early onset of puberty

D. Tall stature

E. Cataracts

21. Diseases associated with an increased risk of malignancy include:

A. Xeroderma pigmentosa

B. Klinefelter's syndrome

C. Neurofibromatosis

D. Coeliac disease

E. Down's syndrome

22. Undescended testes:

A. Is common in preterm babies

B. There is increased risk of malignancy in children

C. Is associated with myotonic dystrophy

D. Is seen in Klinefelter's syndrome

E. There is increased risk of infertility

23. Gilbert syndrome:

A. Is autosomal recessive

B. Presents with conjugated hyperbilirubinaemia

C. Jaundice is exacerbated by alcohol

D. Is more common in females

E. There is higher incidence of breast milk jaundice

24. Down's syndrome is associated with increased incidence of:

A. Coeliac disease

B. Patents ductus arteriosus

C. Hirschsprung's disease

D. Oesophageal atresia

E. Pulmonary hypertension

25. School refusal:

A. Is more common in boys

B. Is associated with depression in up to 70%

C. Separation anxiety may be a contributing factor

D. Is characteristically seen in children with lower ability

E. May be part of a conduct disorder

26. Sleep problems:

A. Maternal anxiety may contribute

B. Improved with sleeping with parents

C. Sedating antihistamines help

D. Nightmares are most common between 5 to 8 years

E. Sleepwalking is most often seen in children aged 5 to 8 years

27. Birthmarks:

A. Strawberry naevi are present at birth

B. Congenital melanocytic naevi are usually more than 5 mm

C. Port wine stains usually disappear in a few months

D. Strawberry naevi are associated with the Sturge-Weber syndrome

E. Salmon patches resolve spontaneously

28. Food allergies and intolerance:

A. Lactose intolerance is usually due to a congenital deficiency of the lactase enzyme

B. Radioallergosorbent testing (RAST) is highly sensitive for diagnosing cow's milk allergy

C. Early onset allergy to peanuts is likely to persist

D. Soya products should not be used in infants less than 6 months

E. Soya milk is recommended in patients with lactose intolerance

29. Foreign body inhalation:

A. They may not be a history of aspiration

B. Bilateral wheeze on clinical examination is common

C. The commonest cause is the peanut which can be seen on chest x-ray

D. The foreign body is usually expectorated and invasive treatment is not required

E. Bronchiectasis is a known complication

30. Umbilical hernia:

A. Must be surgically repaired if not closed by 2 years

B. Usually present at birth

C. Supra- umbilical herniae usually resolve spontaneously

D. There is a higher incidence of strangulation in the older child

E. Is commoner in males

31. Antenatal diagnosis by amniocentesis is possible for:

A. Congenital adrenal hyperplasia

B. Sickle cell disease

C. Duchenne muscular dystrophy

D. Gastroschisis

E. Friedreich's ataxia

32. Long-term complications of intrauterine growth retardation include:

A. Hypertension

B. Diabetes mellitus

C Hyperlipidaemia

D. Epilepsy

E. Asthma

33. Laryngomalacia:

A. Is the most common cause of stridor in the first year of life

B. Stridor improves in the supine position

C. Can lead to faltering growth

D. Is usually associated with respiratory distress

E. Usually resolves by 2 years

34. Cystic hygroma:

A. Can be identified antenatally

B. Diagnosis is on biopsy

C. Treatment is usually by surgical excision

D. Involutes after infection

E. Can cause dysphagia

35. Hypospadias:

A. Incidence is one in 500 live births

B. Is associated with deficient testosterone secretion

C. Should be investigated if associated with undescended testes

D. Can be corrected by circumcision

E. Is usually associated with renal tract anomalies

36. Methylphenidate:

A. Can be started by a GP in a child diagnosed with attention deficit hyperactivity disorder

B. Does not cure ADHD

C. May lead to depression

D. Can lead to hypotension and fainting attacks

E. Side effects include weight gain

37. Poor prognostic signs in acute lymphoblastic leukaemia include:

A. Philadelphia chromosome

B. Age more than 9 years

C. Female sex

D. Caucasian ethnicity

E. Central nervous system disease

38. Vesico-ureteric reflux:

A. Is familial

B. Newborn siblings should be screened

C. Is diagnosed on ultrasound scan

D. Reflux nephropathy leads to renal failure in 50%

E. Long-term antibiotic prophylaxis is needed

39. Causes of hypertension in children:

A. Acute nephritis

B. Congenital adrenal hyperplasia

C. Hypothyroidism

D. Neuroblastoma

E. Ventricular septal defect

40. Myasthenia gravis:

A. Usually presents in the first year

B. Adolescent boys are most commonly affected

C. Bulbar and proximal limb muscles are affected first

D. Extra- ocular muscles are affected later

E. Creatinine kinase may be raised

41. Meningitis in the neonate:

A. Neck stiffness is a classical sign

B. Group B Streptococcus is the most common causative organism

C. Neurological sequelae maybe seen in up to 50%

D. There may be subarachnoid effusions

E. Haemophilus influenza may lead to deafness

42. Vitamin D deficiency:

A. Is seen in prolonged breastfeeding

B. Can be caused by phenytoin

C. Leads to high plasma calcium

D. Is associated with liver disease

E. Primary prevention with vitamins is carried out in the UK

43. White pupillary reflex (leukocoria) may be due to:

A. Cataract

B. Retinoblastoma

C. Glaucoma

D. Retinopathy of prematurity

E. Toxoplasmosis

44. In schizophrenia with childhood onset:

A. Catatonia is common

B. Perinatal difficulties are an implicating factor

C. MRI scan is indicated in a psychotic presentation

D. Acute onset is associated with bad prognosis

E. Younger age at onset is associated with bad prognosis

45. Organic causes of psychosis include:

A. Wilson's disease

B. Systemic lupus erythematosus

C. Epilepsy

D. Vasculitis

E. Prednisolone administration

46. Blistering disorders:

A. Bullous pemphigoid usually lasts for 2 to 4 years

B. Mean age of presentation of dermatitis herpetiformis is at 12 years

C. There is mucous membrane involvement in bullous pemphigoid in 25%

D. Gluten-free diet helps improve the rash in dermatitis herpetiformis

E. Nikolsky's sign is seen in bullous pemphigoid

47. Non-gastrointestinal manifestations of coeliac disease include:

A. Rickets

B. Alopecia

C. Migraine

D. Amenorrhoea

E. Iron deficiency anaemia

48. Developmental dysplasia of the hip (DDH):

A. Is more common in males

B. the Ortolani test involves adducting and depressing the femur

C. Barlow's test is abducting the dislocated hip to reduce it

D. Ortolani's test can be used to reliably detect DDH at 10 weeks

E. Positive Trendelenberg test is seen in the older child

49. Nocturnal enuresis:

A. Can be a sign of maltreatment

B. Lifting and waking can promote long-term dryness

C. Dry bed training with or without an alarm is advisable

D. Desmopressin should be used in a child aged 5 years

E. Oxybutynin is licensed for children over 7 years

50. Meningitis:

A. Meningococcal serogroup C infection remains the most important infectious cause of death in children in the UK

B. Highest incidence is in children less than 2 years old

C. Fatality rate is less than 5%

D. Ciprofloxacin is the first line chemoprophylactic agent

E. Benzylpenicillin should only be given if there is a rash

51. Encopresis:

A. Is defined as the inappropriate passage of faeces usually on the underwear after the age of 7 years

B. Psychiatric disturbance is common

C. Usually persists into adolescence

D. Is associated with hyperthyroidism

E. Maybe a sign of sexual abuse

52. The UK neonatal screening programme:

A. Neonatal blood spots are collected on day 3

B. Guthrie test may be false-negative if on antibiotics

C. Screens for sickle cell disease

D. Screens for Duchenne muscular dystrophy

E. Screens for MCADD (Medium chain acyl-CoA dehydrogenase deficiency)

53. Obesity in children may be due to:

A. Hyperpituitarism

B. Hyperinsulinism

C. Hypergonadism

D. Psychological disturbances

E. Prader- Willi syndrome

54. Parental responsibility:

A. Both biological parents automatically have parental responsibility

B. The father can acquire parental responsibility if he marries the mother

C. The father has parental responsibility if he is unmarried, but his name was registered on the birth certificate before December 2003

D. An unmarried father has parental responsibility if he obtains a residence order

E. Biological parents lose parental responsibility when a child is subject to a care order

55. Screening for Coeliac disease should be considered in the following:

A. Depression

B. Bipolar disorder

C. Persistent abnormal liver function tests

D. Turner syndrome

E. Leukaemia

56. Eating disorders in children:

A. Higher prevalence in lower social class

B. Complications include osteoporosis

C. May have lanugo hair

D. Mortality rate is less than 5%

E. Associated with non-specific EEG abnormalities

57. Increased incidence of surfactant deficiency is seen in:

A. Females

B. Maternal diabetes

C. Maternal opiate use

D. Elective Caesarean section

E. Sepsis

58. Retinoblastoma:

A. Commonly diagnosed at 6 months of age

B. There is a family history of retinoblastoma in 50%

C. May present with a squint

D. There is a 90% percent 5 year survival rate

E. Long-term follow-up is not needed

59. Meningitis:

A. The most common cause of viral meningitis is herpes simplex

B. The cerebrospinal fluid protein level in bacterial meningitis is usually normal or low

C. Neck stiffness is often absent in infants

D. Steroids reduce the severity of deafness

E. Mycobacterium tuberculosis affects older children

60. Enuresis:

A. Diurnal enuresis is much more common in boys

B. Is associated with psychiatric illness in up to 25%

C. Alarms should not be used in children less than 7 years of age

D. Urinalysis should be done routinely in all cases

E. Lifting and waking the child is useful

ANSWERS

Answers Paper 1

The following statements are true.

1. AC

Anorexia nervosa may cause fungal skin infections, reduced metabolic rate, hypokalaemia due to vomiting, increased cortisol and reduced thyroxine levels. Anorexia occurs in one in 100 teenagers. Diagnostic features for anorexia nervosa include: self- induced weight loss of more than 15% bodyweight, through dietary restriction, vomiting, laxative abuse and exercise, which may lead to stunting of growth. There is intense fear of gaining weight, even when underweight, and abnormal perception of bodyweight and image, with a feeling of being fat, and amenorrhoea.

2. ABDE

There may be increased pulmonary vascular markings on chest x-ray in atrial septal defect. Cardiomegaly is seen on chest x-ray in 60% of children with large ventricular septal defects, and is seen as early as the age of two months. There are oligaemic lung fields on chest x-ray in tetralogy of Fallot. The ECG shows partial right bundle branch block in up to 90% of cases with atrial septal defects. Rib notching may be seen on chest x-ray in coarctation of the aorta due to development of large intercostal arteries running under the ribs posteriorly to bypass the obstruction.

3. DE

Separation anxiety is seen from six months of age and peaks at 15 months. Stranger anxiety is seen from nine months and peaks at two years. School phobia is common in social classes one and two. Fear of nightmares is seen in children up to 11 years of age, and is most common between 3 to 5 years of age. 1/3 of children with school phobia will have adults neuroses especially Agoraphobia.

4. BCDE

Bronchiectasis is associated with hypogammaglobulinaemia and alpha-1 antitrypsin deficiency. It may occur after a foreign body inhalation and after infections such as measles and pertussis. Cyanosis maybe present in severe cases. It can occur after childhood pneumonia and chronic lung disease of prematurity.

5. ACD

Cystic fibrosis is associated with nasal polyps. Diabetes is found in 10% of teenage cases. Neonatal screening is available with immunoreactive trypsin. It has a carrier rate of 1:25, leading to disease in one in 2500 live births in white babies. The gene responsible is autosomal recessive and encodes the cystic fibrosis transmembrane conductance regulator

(CFTR), and is on chromosome 7. In the UK 60% are homozygous for the delta F08 mutation. Asthma co-exists in 20% of children. In the UK, all babies are screened for cystic fibrosis as part of the newborn screening program since October 2007, with the Guthrie test.

6. BCDE

Side-effects of methylphenidate include anorexia and weight loss, insomnia, tics, psychosis, hypertension and it lowers seizure threshold. It is used for the treatment of attention deficit hyperactivity disorder (ADHD) and should be started by child psychiatrists or paediatricians with expertise in ADHD. Height, weight, pulse and blood pressure should be monitored at least six monthly. GPs may agree to share care. Drug treatment does not cure ADHD; however it improves the symptoms to allow other interventions. It is not licensed for children less than six years.

7. AC

Neglect is the commonest form of child abuse. Mortality in children attributable to abuse and neglect is reported to be 200 deaths per annum by OFSTED, which is about three deaths per week (OFSTED 2008). This is higher than the NSPCC's estimate of at least a child a week; this is because the NSPCC has traditionally relied on the home office data on homicide. In Britain one in 1000 children suffers severe physical abuse. Boys are more likely to be on the child protection register up to the age of 10. Sexual abuse often begins under the age of three years.

8. BCDE

Skeletal survey should be done in any child with suspected physical abuse especially if less than three years of age, in soft tissue injury in an older child, non-accidental injury especially fractures. Coma, a child dying in suspicious unusual circumstances, unexplained neurological symptoms including apnoea, seizures, reduced consciousness, intracranial injury with the absence of history of significant accidental trauma. It is to be considered as part of investigation of siblings where abuse has been identified in another child in the family unit. It may need to be repeated if the first survey was negative, a bone scan is not available and bony injury is suspected. Bone scan should be considered particularly if bony injury is suspected but not confirmed on initial skeletal survey.

9. BCD

Prolonged QT syndrome usually presents in the first decade. On electrocardiogram, the QT interval is more than 440ms. It is associated with syncope during exercise, stress or emotion. It can be caused by various medications such as certain antihistamines, domperidone, cisapride and some anti-depressants.

10. BC

A police protection order lasts for 72 hours. An Emergency Protection Order lasts for eight days and can be extended for another seven days. It may be granted by court if there is reasonable cause to believe that the child is likely to suffer harm if not removed from their current accommodation or if there is lack of access on enquiries by the local authority. A Child assessment order may be used if there is a persistent but non- urgent risk of harm. It lasts for up to 7 days. It overrides the objections of a parent to whatever assessment is needed. It also overrides the objection of a child who is of sufficient understanding to make an informed decision. A Supervision order lasts for one year. It gives social services the power and duty to visit the family and to ensure attendance at clinic, nursery, school or hospital visits. A supervision order may be extended for up to 3 years up to the child's 18th birthday.

11. AB

In the social services child protection process, a strategy meeting should take place within seven days and be chaired by a social worker. The initial child protection case conference should be held within 15 working days of the strategy meeting, and should be held within 35 days or sooner of the case referral. The child is placed on the child protection register at the initial child protection case conference. Child protection review is carried out six monthly.

12. ABC

In the neonatal period, cystic fibrosis commonly presents with a positive new born screening test. Some babies present with meconium ileus and bowel obstruction, which may be seen antenatally on an ultrasound scan as hyper -echogenic bowel. Cystic fibrosis may present with obstructive jaundice, steatorrhoea, hypoalbuminaemia, oedema and anaemia, or bleeding from vitamin K deficiency. Cough, frequent chesty episodes and wheeze may be missed as viral infections. Nasal polyps may occur in up to 30%. 99% of males are infertile due to obstruction and abnormal development of the vas deferens, and females may be subfertile.

13. ABCDE

Snoring in children becomes a problem when it is in association with periods of ineffective breathing lasting longer than 15 seconds i.e. obstructive sleep apnoea. The most common cause of obstructive sleep apnoea is adenotonsillar hypertrophy. It is commonly seen in children with Down's syndrome and may be present in the Pierre Robin sequence due to cleft palate and micrognathia. It leads to daytime somnolence and may cause poor growth. If severe it may lead to pulmonary hypertension and cor- pulmonale due to hypoxia and hypercapnia.

14. BC

A long PR interval of more than 0.16 seconds is seen in atrioventricular canal defects; digoxin toxicity associated with short QT, flat or reversed tick appearance of the T waves. Hyperkalaemia is associated with tall peaked T waves. Wolff – Parkinson- White syndrome is associated with a short PR interval

15. D

Whooping cough is a common infection in the UK and is seen with epidemics in winter. It is a notifiable disease. Bordetella pertussis transmission is by droplets and the incubation period is 7 to 14 days. Bronchopneumonia due to secondary bacterial infection is the most common complication and the most common cause of death. Other complications include lobar or segmental collapse, subconjunctival haemorrhage, epistaxis, fitting and nervous system damage. Bronchiectasis is a long-term complication. Clinical diagnosis is confirmed by serological testing, lymphocytosis of up to 20,000/mm3 and immunofluorescent staining from nasopharyngeal swabs, which is positive in 50 to 80% of cases.

16. D

The arms are more affected in spastic diplegia than the legs. Hand preference under the age of one is abnormal, and signifies hemiparesis. In hemiplegia the affected limb may initially be flaccid and hypotonic, but then tone increases. The arm is affected more than the leg. It often presents at 4 to 12 months of age with fisting of the affected hand, a pronated flexed forearm, or tiptoe walk, toe - heel gait on the affected side. Quadriplegia is often associated with learning impairment and seizures. There may be a history of severe hypoxic ischaemia at birth. The trunk is often involved with extensor posturing and poor head control.

17. DE

Prevalence is the proportion of a defined group having a disease at any one time. Incidence is the proportion of a defined group developing a disease within a stated period. 70% of all childhood deaths occur in the first year in England and Wales, and 40% are in the first month. Prevalence is useful when measuring chronic conditions, whereas incidence measures the rate of occurrence of new cases.

18. AE

Stillbirth rate is the number of infants born dead with a gestational age of 24 weeks per 1000 births; in the

UK it is 4.7 per 1000 births, according to the Office for National Statistics (ONS). Perinatal mortality rate is the number of stillbirths and deaths during the first week of life per 1000 total births; in the UK it is 6.6 per 1000 births. Early neonatal mortality rate is the number of deaths at up to 6 days of life per 1000 live births; in the UK it is 2.6 per 1000 live births. Neonatal mortality rate is the number of deaths up to 28 days of life per 1000 live births; this figure for the UK is 2.5 per 1000 live births. Perinatal and neonatal mortality rates are adjusted by excluding terminations of pregnancy and babies born at 22 weeks gestation. Infant mortality rate is the number of deaths in infants under one year of age per 1000 live births this was 3.6 in 1000 in the UK, as per the ONS: Childhood mortality in England and Wales 2014, released April 2016.

19. ABC

Major causes of neonatal mortality are related to prematurity, and infant mortality is to do with perinatal problems associated with prematurity and congenital anomalies. Injury and poisoning are the major causes of death after one year of age. Mortality rates are higher for boys, due to unintentional injury. The ratio of males to females is 1.4:1. Mortality rates are higher in social classes four and five.

20. BDE

Cross-sectional studies determine the prevalence of disease, and may give clues about causation. They examine at the same time an outcome of disease, and the presence of a risk factor. Cohort studies are prospective and give estimation of incidence, they observe over time the effect of exposure to a risk factor or disease in a study cohort in a suitable control group not exposed to the factor or disease. They provide stronger evidence of causation. Case-control studies are done retrospectively, and are useful for studying rare diseases. They are particularly prone to bias; their evidence for causation is weak.

21. CE

Sensitivity is the number of people with the condition who are correctly identified by the test, whereas specificity is the number of people without the condition who are correctly identified by the test. Positive predictive value is the number of positive screening results that are correct i.e. it is the proportion of all those with a positive test result who truly have the disease. The predictive value of a positive result falls as the prevalence declines. Low specificity leads to lots of false positives and has implications for cost effectiveness.

22. CD

Haemophilus influenza B vaccine is non-live, and made from bacterial capsular antigens. Only one vaccine is required if over one year old and not immune. Routine immunisation is recommended up to 4 years. Haemophilus influenza B may cause cellulitis, pericarditis, pneumonia, septic arthritis and osteomyelitis. It can be given if there is a history of prolonged jaundice.

23. ABC

Complications of mumps include; meningoencephalitis, pancreatitis, nephritis, myocarditis, arthritis, deafness, thyroiditis, orchitis and oophoritis. Rubella may cause myocarditis thrombocytopenia arthritis and arthralgia. Complications of measles include; otitis media, laryngitis, bronchitis, myocarditis, encephalomyelitis occurs in one in 1000 cases, and sub-acute sclerosing pan- encephalitis which may occur up to 7 years after measles infection. There is a 10% failure rate from primary vaccination with MMR at 12 to 18 months of age. Rubella infection peaks in the 4-9 year age group.

24. ABCDE

Adverse reactions to the MMR include; malaise, fever, rash within 7 to 10 days which is not infectious, and is a mini- measles reaction. Parotid swelling in 1%, febrile convulsions one in 1000, encephalopathy, thrombocytopenia which is rare and occurs, one in 20,000 and usually has a spontaneous resolution. Arthropathy is rare and may be due to the rubella component. MMR is contraindicated in children who are allergic to neomycin or kanamycin.

25. CE

Babies born to mothers who are Hepatitis B surface antigen positive and have the e- antigen antibody should have the vaccine only, however if the baby weighs 1.5 kg or less, they should receive the immunoglobulin as well. If the mother is hepatitis B surface antigen positive and hepatitis B e- antigen positive, the baby should be vaccinated as well as receive immunoglobulin at birth. Further doses are recommended at one month, two months and 12 months of age. Hepatitis B surface antigen testing is carried out at 12 months of age. Booster vaccine is given at five years of age.

26. AC

Visual impairment is defined as corrected acuity of less than 6/18 in the better eye; it may not be correctable after five years of age. In amblyopia, the defect is not correctable by glasses. About 45% of cases of visual loss are of genetic origin. The defect is most commonly in the cerebral and visual pathways in up to 50%. The retina is involved in up to 30 % of cases.

27. E

Squints occur in approximately 4% of children. They are common in newborn, occurring in up to 70% at 1 month, reducing to 50 % in 2 month old babies. There is a strong familial incidence. A squint is a misalignment of the visual axis of one eye. To prevent double vision, the image from the squinting eye is suppressed by the brain. Without treatment, this can lead to amblyopia. A squint is either latent which is only present at certain times, such as tiredness, stress or illness; or manifest, which is present all the time. In a latent squint, there is movement of the covered eye on uncovering. In a manifest squint, there is movement of the uncovered eye on covering. The cover test is performed at 30 cm distance. Alternating squints are very common and have a good prognosis. In an alternating squint, the patient uses either eye for fixation while the other eye deviates, as both eyes are being used vision develops well; as opposed to monocular squints, where only one eye is used to fixate and the other deviates, which leads to amblyopia as the deviated eye is not being used.

28. CE

1-2 children per 1000 population have permanent childhood deafness. 84% is congenital and 16% acquired. The prevalence of congenital sensorineural hearing loss is 1 to 2 per 1000, and conductive hearing loss is 4 to 11 in 100. Pendred's syndrome is associated with a sensorineural hearing loss and Treacher-Collin's syndrome is associated with conductive hearing loss. A stay of 48 hours in the neonatal intensive care unit increases the risk of hearing loss. Middle ear disease may produce conductive hearing loss of 30 dB.

29. ABDE

The neonatal screening tests used to identify deafness, are the evoked otoacoustic emissions test (OAE) and the auditory brainstem response test. The evoked otoacoustic emissions test checks the cochlear pathways and measures the function of the inner ear. In a healthy cochlea, vibration of the hair cells in response to noise generates acoustic energy called otoacoustic emissions. The automated auditory brainstem response test is done for babies in special care. It measures the integrity of the inner ear and the auditory pathway. Electrophysiological response from the brainstem is detected by scalp electrodes. The distraction test is done at 7 to 9 months of age. The co-operative language test is done at 18 months to 2 years of age. 50 dB is required for normal speech to develop. The school sweep test is used as a screening test at the pre-school entry. It is quicker to perform because various sound frequencies are tested at only one intensity. If the child fails at any frequency, then full audiometry is performed. Pure tone audiometry can be done on a child from the age of four years.

30. BDE

Behavioural problems are associated with low parental IQ. Marital discord leads to internalising behaviour in girls and externalising behaviour in boys. Boys are more vulnerable to behavioural problems than girls. Behavioural problems are more common in children with low IQ and those living in high rise housing.

31. ABD

Tuberous sclerosis is a dominantly inherited disorder with variable expression. More than 50 per cent of cases of Tuberous sclerosis are sporadic. It is characterised by skin and nervous system abnormalities, and may present with infantile spasms or epilepsy in up to 95%. Up to 60 to 80 % have renal involvement with enlarged kidneys, most commonly due to angiomyolipomata or polycystic kidneys. Adenoma sebaceum is seen over the nose and cheeks in a butterfly distribution, rarely under the age of two years, but in more than 50% by five years, and increases with age.

32. ABC

Neurofibromatosis type I accounts for 90% of cases, and is associated with an increased incidence of Wilm's tumour and phaeochromocytoma. Type II generally presents in the second decade, and is associated with bilateral acoustic neuromas and other nervous system tumours, like gliomas and meningioma. Lisch nodules are seen in Type 1.

33. DE

The incidence of Tuberous sclerosis is one in 50,000. There are at least two separate genes that cause tuberous sclerosis, on chromosomes 9 and 16. Intracranial calcification is seen in 50%. Multiple intracranial gliotic hamartomas and nodules may undergo malignant change. Ash- leaf spots are hypomelanotic macules, which may be present at birth and increase during childhood and usually persist throughout life. In fair skinned races, they are only visible with a Wood's lamp, using ultraviolet light to make them stand out. Shagreen patches are areas of thick leathery skin, like orange –peel, and are usually seen on the lumbosacral region or back of the neck. Retinal phacomata may be seen near the optic disc as dense white areas due to local degeneration.

34. ABCE

Inguinal hernia result due to the persistence of the patent processes vaginalis, which is a peritoneal sac along the path of testicular descent into the scrotum. Inguinal hernias are present in 9 to 11% of preterm babies; the incidence in the general population is 1 to 2%, and is 10 times more common in boys. 15% are bilateral. Girls presenting with inguinal hernia should have their chromosomes checked, due to a rare association of inguinal hernia in girls with complete androgen insensitivity syndrome. Irreducibility can lead to obstruction which may present as abdominal pain, distension, vomiting and lead to strangulation, therefore elective repair is advised. Hydrocoeles usually present as symptomless fluid- filled swellings of the scrotum that are trans- illuminable. They may present as tense swellings during an acute illness. Most hydrocoeles resolve without surgery in the first year of life, and should be operated on if they persist after two years. They may be associated with a tumour.

35. ABD

Prader-Willi syndrome is associated with failure to thrive in infancy and difficulty in feeding; however, later there is obesity due to hyperphagia. There may be undescended testes and cryptorchidism. It is associated with short stature. The genetic defect arises from the deletion of the paternally derived long arm of chromosome 15 q in 70 % of cases, whereas the absence of maternal contribution to chromosome 15 leads to Angelman's syndrome.

36. ABC

Prader- Willi syndrome is associated with breech presentation, neonatal hypotonia and feeding difficulties in the newborn period. There is a tendency to diabetes mellitus and obesity. Hypogonadism and strabismus are also seen. There may be congenital dislocation of the hips. IQ is reduced to usually 40-70. Behavioural problems such as temper-tantrums, food-seeking behaviour and obsessional traits are seen. Inappropriate laughter is seen in Angelman's syndrome.

37. BDE

Phimosis is the narrowing of the prepuce that prevents retraction of the foreskin. The prepuce is normally non-retractile at birth and early childhood. Pathological phimosis is most commonly due to Balanitis Xerotica Obliterans (BXO), in which the foreskin is thickened, inflamed and scarred, and needs surgical treatment, with circumcision. BXO affects 2% of boys by the age of 17 years and is very rare in those aged under five years. In paraphimosis the prepuce retracts and becomes stuck behind the glans. The glans becomes swollen and oedematous; it needs reduction under general anaesthesia and follow up with circumcision maybe needed later to prevent recurrence. 1% of 17 year olds have non-retractile foreskins which do not need treatment.

38. BD

The differential diagnosis of the acute scrotum in childhood includes; testicular torsion, torted Hydatid of Morgagni, epididymo-orchitis, testicular trauma and idiopathic scrotal oedema. Testicular torsion must be excluded in a child with acute scrotal pain. Peak incidence is around 10 to 12 years of age, but it can occur at any age. It usually presents with sudden, severe scrotal pain, often associated with nausea and vomiting. The scrotum may be red and oedematous. Testicular torsion is a surgical emergency. The contralateral testes should also be fixed. It may be difficult to differentiate it with torsion of the Hydatid of Morgagni, in which the onset of pain is gradual and there is localised tenderness at the upper pole of the testis with a blue dot sign. Orchitis is rare in post-pubertal boys and presents with fever and testicular pain. In children, epididymo- orchitis is usually associated with a urinary tract infection, as the infected urine refluxes down the vas. Idiopathic scrotal oedema is commonest in 1 to 3 year olds. The child is well and afebrile, the scrotal skin is cellulitic but the testes are not tender. It usually settles spontaneously within a few days.

39. ACE

Pyloric stenosis occurs in 2-3 per 1000 live births. It is commoner in males, with a male to female ratio of 4:1. It results due to hypertrophy of the pyloric muscle, leading to gastric outlet obstruction. The cause remains unknown; however there may be a strong family history in some cases, particularly in girls. It presents with non-bilious, projectile vomiting, most commonly at 4 to 6 weeks of life. It may lead to weight loss and dehydration, and maybe misdiagnosed as gastro-oesophageal reflux. Constipation is common due to reduced fluid intake. There may be visible peristalsis, and the diagnostic sign is a palpable pyloric tumour, felt as an olive-shaped mass just above and to the right of the umbilicus during a test feed. Ultrasound may be done to confirm the diagnosis .Treatment is by surgical correction.

40. BCD

Intussusception is the telescoping of the intestine. It commonly occurs in boys, with a male to female ratio of 4:1 and peaks at 5 to 9 months of age. Incidence is one in 500 children. It commonly occurs in association with viral gastroenteritis, due to enlarged Peyer's patches. In 5 to 10% there may be a pathological lead point, for example a polyp or Meckel's diverticulum. It classically presents with, abdominal pain with drawing up of the legs, bleeding per rectum, with "redcurrant jelly stools", there may be a palpable abdominal mass. Vomiting, constipation or diarrhoea may be present. Patients can present with signs of shock and sepsis. Fever is due to necrosis of bowel and sepsis. Abdominal x-ray shows signs of small bowel obstruction and soft tissue opacity. Ultrasound scan confirms the diagnosis. Treatment is by pneumatic reduction which has a 50 to 75% success rate, or by surgery. There is a recurrence rate of about 10%.

41. ADE

Spina bifida occurs due to defects in the fusion of the dorsal vertebral bodies. It most commonly occurs in the lumbosacral region. Meningocoele is the herniation of the meninges and fluid with a skin covering; it requires surgical closure, prognosis is excellent. A Myelomeningocoele is the herniation of spinal neural tissue which may or may not be covered by meninges or skin. There is usually abnormal neurology and is commonly associated with a hydrocephalus. Treatment is by surgical closure and prognosis is related to the severity of associated problems.

42. ABCDE

The overall incidence of neural tube defects has decreased, because of antenatal screening and maternal supplementation with folic acid, from preconception to 12 weeks gestation. It can be diagnosed antenatally by raised alpha-fetoprotein and ultrasound scan. Ventriculo- peritoneal shunt may be required for hydrocephalus. There may be associated bladder or bowel dysfunction, such as rectal prolapse, renal tract anomalies like hypospadias, horse-shoe kidneys, congenital heart disease and craniofacial anomalies.

43. CE

Noonan syndrome is an autosomal dominant condition, with 50% caused by mutation on chromosome 12. Features of Noonan syndrome include, short stature and cardiac defects in up to 80 % such as, pulmonary stenosis, atrial and ventricular septal defects and hypertrophic cardiomyopathy. The cardiac defects in Noonan syndrome are predominantly right-sided, whereas in Turner's syndrome are mostly left-sided, for example coarctation and aortic stenosis .There may be broad neck, chest deformities, cryptorchidism, and mild developmental delay. Mild learning disability is seen in 30 %. Typical facial features include epicanthic folds, ptosis, low set ears, trident hairline posteriorly and hypertelorism.

44. ABCE

Pierre- Robin sequence has a sporadic inheritance but may be familial. It is characterised by 3 features; micrognathia, glossoptosis or protruding tongue, and cleft palate. The large tongue may obstruct the airway causing apnoea particularly during sleep, prone- positioning may help but occasionally tracheostomy is required. There is mandibular hypoplasia.

45. CDE

Cerebral palsy is a disorder of tone, posture or movement, due to a static lesion affecting the developing nervous system. At least 80% of cases of cerebral palsy are due to prenatally acquired causes.

About 7% are related to intra-partum asphyxia. Epilepsy is present in 25% with hemiplegia. Mental retardation may be present in up to 50% of children with hemiplegia, whereas intellectual function is mostly preserved in spastic diplegia.

46. ABCE

Spastic quadriplegia is associated with damage to the brain stem. It is caused by disruption to the spinal reflex arc by the upper motor neuron. It affects all the skeletal muscles and causes increased tone and reflexes, clasp- knife phenomenon, plantar flexion, the hip, wrist and elbow are flexed, shoulder is adducted. Bulbar muscles may be spastic, giving rise to feeding problems, reflux and breathing difficulties. The overall incidence of cerebral palsy has increased in the last 20 years due to the increased number of survivors of neonatal care.

47. ABD

Puberty starts on average at the age of 10 years in girls and 12 years in boys. In boys, the first sign of puberty is the increase in growth of the testes and scrotum, and later by development of pubic hair and penile growth. Peak growth velocity in boys occurs with testicular volumes of 10 to 12 ml. In girls, the first signs of puberty are the appearance of the breast bud and breast development. Peak growth velocity in girls is at breast development stage 2 to 3. Menarche occurs at breast stage 4. Precocious puberty is rare and usually pathological in boys and needs to be investigated. Precocious puberty is commoner in girls with a female to male ratio of 10:1. It is usually benign but needs to be monitored. Delayed puberty is commoner in boys.

48. BD

About 10% of childhood epilepsy is due to absence seizures or Petit- mal epilepsy as it was previously called. This is characterised by brief episodes, lasting 5 to 20 seconds of staring, during which the child is unaware of their surroundings. There is a 3 hertz spike wave activity on the electroencephalogram, which can be brought on by hyperventilation. Valproate is the drug of choice in generalised epilepsy such as tonic- clonic seizures, absences and myoclonic seizures. Infantile spasms occur commonly from the age of three months to one year, peaking at 4 to 6 months. Infantile spasms or Salam attacks, involve brief sudden muscular contractions of the trunk, leading to flexion and extension of the body. There is disorganised activity on the electroencephalogram, described as hypsarrhythmia. It may be idiopathic, or symptomatic; due to physical causes, like tuberous sclerosis or perinatal hypoxic injury. Treatment is with steroids or Vigabatrin. Prognosis depends on the cause; generally children with idiopathic causes do better than the symptomatic group which may continue to have seizures in 90% of cases. It is associated with developmental delay and regression.

49. AB

Typically absence seizures present during the first decade and 95% of children will have remission in adolescence. Infantile spasm is associated with learning disabilities in most children in the symptomatic group with underlying pathology. Juvenile myoclonic epilepsy is twice as common in females, and usually presents between the ages of 10 to 20 years. Myoclonic jerks classically occur within the first hour of awakening. There is high risk of generalised tonic - clonic seizures. Benign rolandic epilepsy is a common form of benign epilepsy in childhood, and comprises 10 to 20 per cent of all epilepsies. The classic presentation of this condition is predominantly nocturnal sensorimotor seizures with onset in one side of the face or a hand, spreading down and may generalise into tonic clonic seizures. Electroencephalogram shows rolandic spike waves in the centro- temporal area. It is associated with fits in the first decade which generally stop in the mid-teens.

50. DE

Febrile convulsions occur in 3% of children between the age of six months and five years. There is a 30% risk of recurrence overall, and 50% recurrence in children less than one year of age. The absolute risk of a non-febrile seizure after one febrile convulsion is one to 5%. 10 to 20% have relatives with a seizure disorder indicating that there may be a genetic predisposition. If prolonged, may cause temporal and hippocampal sclerosis and gliosis, which may lead to temporal lobe epilepsy in later childhood or adolescence.

51. BCDE

Sodium valproate may cause nausea, abdominal pain, weight gain and increased appetite. It may cause transient hair loss, thrombocytopenia and liver dysfunction. Carbamazepine may cause leukopenia, thrombocytopenia, a lupus- like syndrome with a rash and ataxia. Vigabatrin may cause sedation and restriction in peripheral visual fields. It is used in partial seizures and for infantile spasms.

52. ABCDE

Achondroplasia is autosomal dominant but there are new mutations in 80 % of cases. It is seen in one in 20,000 births. It is associated with shortening of the proximal limbs, short fingers and toes, trident hand, recurrent otitis media and conductive or sensorineural deafness. There may be kyphosis, spinal cord compression and hydrocephalus.

53. BC

Cornelia de Lange syndrome is a rare syndrome with an incidence of one in 50,000 live births. Inheritance is sporadic. There is intrauterine and postnatal growth impairment leading to short stature, limb anomalies and hirsutism. The distinctive facial features include arched eyebrows, short upturned nose, and thin lips with downturned corners of the mouth. There may be abnormal genitalia, undescended testes and hypospadias. Cornelia de Lange syndrome is associated with microcephaly, seizures, congenital heart disease and mental retardation. Limb malformation is seen in 25% of cases and includes micromelia, oligodactyly, clinodactyly and proximal implantation of the thumbs.

54. AC

Ewing's sarcoma occurs in boys more commonly than girls, and in the 5 to 20 year age group. It usually presents as an infection, with fever, localised swelling, heat, and redness. It occurs in the diaphysis of long bones, commonly the pelvis, femur, ribs and humerus. The white blood cells and ESR are raised. X-ray shows onion skin layers of periosteal bone formation. Metastasis occurs early to the lungs and other bones. Biopsy is needed for diagnosis. Treatment is with radiotherapy and chemotherapy. The 5 year survival rate is 55%.

55. CDE

The prevalence of Angelman syndrome is one in 10 to 20,000. In 80% of cases there is a deletion on the maternal chromosome 15. It is associated with microcephaly, severe learning disability, ataxia, hypotonia, seizures and optic atrophy. There is unprovoked laughter and clapping, and characteristic arm posture like a puppet. There may be widely spaced teeth and a prominent jaw.

56. BE

Fragile X syndrome causes learning disability, autism and seizures. The inheritance is X- linked. The fragile site is located on the distal long arm of chromosome X. All males and around 50% of females with the full mutation are affected, though females are typically less severely affected. It is associated with a large head with prominent forehead, thickening of the nasal bridge, prominent jaw, large posteriorly rotated ears and pale blue eye irides. There is macro-orchidism and hyperkinetic behaviour. Female carriers have a higher risk of around 50% of premature ovarian failure or early menopause. Clinical manifestations relate to the expansion of the tri-nucleotide repeat sequence, and increasing severity of the condition is seen with increased expansion. The tri-nucleotide expansion increases with each generation.

57. ACDE

Kallmann's syndrome or hypogonadotrophic hypogonadism and anosmia, arises due to a defect in the migration of gonadotropin releasing hormone releasing neurons and olfactory neurons that occurs during early fetal development. It is an X-linked condition which may be autosomal dominant or recessive. It is characterised by synkinesia, which is mirror image movements, congenital renal anomalies, including unilateral renal agenesis, undescended testes, and increased risk of testicular tumours, micro-penis and obesity.

58. AC

Kallmann's syndrome is associated with choanal atresia and cleft palate. Deafness is occasionally present. The serum testosterone level is low and prepubertal levels of gonadotropins. Treatment is with testosterone replacement and pulsatile gonadotropin releasing hormone.

59. BC

50 % of children with Down's syndrome have a congenital heart defect. The commonest being atrioventricular septal defects, but ventricular septal defects, and atrial septal defects may occur separately. Noonan syndrome is associated with hypertrophic obstructive cardiomyopathy and pulmonary stenosis. Pulmonary stenosis is the commonest heart defect seen in William's syndrome

and supra- valvular aortic stenosis. 8% of cases of congenital heart disease are associated with major chromosomal abnormalities. It is usually associated with anomalies of the kidneys, vertebra or the limbs. The overall infant cardiac surgical mortality rate has been reduced to 5%; it was up to 20% in the 70s.

60. CDE

Tetralogy of Fallot comprises of ventricular septal defect, pulmonary stenosis, overriding aorta and right ventricular hypertrophy. It is usually asymptomatic and rarely presents with severe cyanosis at birth, which worsens as the child gets older. It is commonly diagnosed at 4 to 6 weeks of age. Most cases have elective repair at 6 to 9 months; however 10% may require a BT shunt sooner if severely cyanosed. The electrocardiogram is usually normal at birth but shows right ventricular hypertrophy when older. Chest x-ray is usually normal, but may show a boot-shaped heart with an upturned apex and reduced vascular margins. It may lead to cerebral abscess and thrombosis, bacterial endocarditis and haemorrhagic tendency. It is associated with Goldenhar and Down's syndrome.

Answers Paper 2

The following statements are true.

1. AB

Transposition of the great arteries involves a connection between the aorta and the right ventricle, and the pulmonary artery with the left ventricle. This condition is not compatible with life, unless if there is mixing of the blood from both circulations via a septal defect. It usually presents with cyanosis in the first few hours to days of life. The electrocardiogram is normal. Chest x-ray may be normal, with increased pulmonary vascular markings and egg- on- side appearance of the cardiac shadow, due to the antero- posterior relationship of the great vessels and hypertrophied right ventricle. The child may need resuscitation, and arterial switch operation is carried out in the first few weeks of life.

2. ABCE

Medical complications of anorexia include hypokalaemia, hypochloraemic metabolic alkalosis, oedema, renal calculi and renal failure. Parotitis, delayed gastric emptying and constipation. Anorexia may cause bradycardia, hypotension, arrhythmias and rarely cardiomyopathy. Other complications include; dental caries, periodontitis, reversible cortical atrophy, non-specific EEG changes, carotinaemia, reduced bone density and amenorrhoea.

3. ABCDE

Prolonged QT syndrome is characterised by abnormal ventricular repolarisation and arrhythmias. It may be misdiagnosed as epilepsy and there is an association with a risk of sudden death. Genetic testing is available; it can be autosomal dominant or recessive. It may be associated with congenital deafness.

4. ABCDE

Differential diagnosis of physical abuse includes: copper deficiency; blood disorders such as idiopathic thrombocytopenic purpura need to be excluded. Impetigo needs to be differentiated from burns and scalds. Rickets may be confused with fractures in which case, blood tests for vitamin D and bone profile is needed. Osteogenesis imperfecta, though rare has to be considered and osteomyelitis especially in fractures, a white cell count and blood cultures are useful. Severe accidental injury should be considered and highlights the importance of meticulous history taking. Retinal haemorrhages and subdural haemorrhages may occur after birth but usually resolve within the neonatal period.

5. BCDE

Innocent murmurs are functional or physiological heart murmurs, which occur in 40% of all children.

The heart is structurally normal. Innocent murmurs are soft, systolic and short; are heard over the left sternal edge, and the child is asymptomatic. Still's murmur may be confused with a ventricular septal defect murmur. It is heard in the midst to lower left sternal edge and reduces in the upright posture. Venous hum is heard at the upper sternal edge and disappears by gentle compression or on lying flat. It may be confused with a patent ductus arteriosus. Pulmonary flow murmur is frequently seen in preterm neonates.

6. ABC

The incidence of congenital heart disease is five to eight per 1000 live births. Maternal diabetes may lead to transposition of the great arteries and Truncus arteriosus in the baby. Noonan's syndrome is associated with hypertrophic obstructive cardiomyopathy and pulmonary stenosis. Antenatal rubella infection is associated with patent ductus arteriosus and pulmonary stenosis in the baby. Children with Di George's syndrome should not have live vaccines.

7. ABD

In the normal neonatal ECG, there are dominant R waves in V1 and deep S waves in V6. Persisting neonatal RS progression after the first month implies right ventricular hypertrophy, as is seen in tetralogy of

Fallot, pulmonary stenosis and pulmonary hypertension. PR interval in children is 0.08 to 0.16 seconds, which are 2 to 4 little squares. A long PR interval is seen in atrioventricular septal defects, myocarditis, digoxin toxicity, hyperkalaemia, hypothermia, and Diphtheria and Duchenne muscular dystrophy. A short PR interval is seen in Wolff-Parkinson White syndrome and Pompe's disease. A short PR interval predisposes to supraventricular tachyarrhythmias. The normal QT interval is less than 0.4 seconds. A long QT interval is seen in: hypocalcaemia, hypokalaemia, hypomagnesaemia, hypothermia, Romano Ward's syndrome, head injury and medication such as domperidone or erythromycin. A long QT predisposes to ventricular tachyarrhythmias.

8. ABCDE

Whooping cough may lead to pneumonia and lobar collapse, epistaxis and subconjunctival haemorrhages. It may lead to convulsions due to hypoxia and may result in cerebral haemorrhages and encephalopathy.

9. BCDE

In Friedreich's ataxia, muscle tone is usually normal or decreased, with weakness. There is associated visual and hearing loss. Cardiac involvement is present in 90% of cases, with atrial fibrillation and hypertrophic cardiomyopathy. Age of onset is usually 8-15 years. There may be cerebellar dysfunction with dysarthria and dysdiadochokinesia.

10. BCDE

Nitric oxide is a vasodilator, and it inhibits platelet aggregation. Its half-life is 3 to 6 seconds, and it is inactivated by haemoglobin. Inhaled nitric oxide causes selective pulmonary vasodilation and is useful in persistent pulmonary hypertension of the new born.

11. BD

In Eisenmenger's syndrome, blood flow through an original left to right shunt, caused by a congenital heart defect becomes reversed, as a result of reactive pulmonary hypertension. Deoxygenated blood is mixed with systemic blood causing cyanosis. It is usually seen with ventricular septal defects, atrioventricular septal defects and patent ductus arteriosus. There is excessive pulmonary blood flow and increased pulmonary vascular resistance. Patients with pulmonary atresia and pulmonary stenosis are protected as there is limited blood flow. It rarely evolves until the second decade.

12. ABD

Patent ductus arteriosus is uncommon in babies born at term after 1 to 2 days. It usually presents in the first few days of life in very low birth weight and premature infants, with a systolic murmur. There is a continuous machinery murmur at the left sternal border, bounding pulses, wide pulse pressure and possibly signs of cardiac failure. It does not usually cause cyanosis except in the presence of pulmonary hypertension. Early treatment with indomethacin has been shown to reduce the risk of necrotising enterocolitis and chronic lung disease. If it persists in the young child, closure is recommended to prevent risk of bacterial endocarditis.

13. BCE

Marfan's syndrome is an autosomal dominant condition, resulting from mutations in the fibrillin gene on chromosome 15. Prevalence is one in 10,000. Clinical features associated with Marfan's syndrome include upward subluxation of the lens, strabismus, myopia and retinal detachment, pneumothorax and chest wall deformities; such as pectus excavatum, carinatum, scoliosis and learning disabilities.

14. ABCDE

Systemic hypertension in children may be due to renal artery stenosis, coarctation of the aorta, vasculitis, polycystic kidney disease, increased steroids; iatrogenic or endogenous, hyperthyroidism, tumours such as

Neuroblastoma and Wilm's tumour, and lead, thallium or mercury poisoning.

15. BD

William's syndrome usually has a sporadic inheritance and is due to a micro-deletion involving the elastin gene on chromosome 7. It is associated with short stature, elfin features, serrated teeth, carp- shaped mouth, hypertelorism and stellate iris. Most have mild to moderate mental retardation with poor visio- spatial skills. It is associated with hypertension.

16. ACDE

About 15% of infants with William's syndrome have hypercalcaemia. There may be enamel hypoplasia and dental mal-occlusion, depressed nasal bridge and broad maxilla with full cheeks. There is aortic stenosis; most commonly supra-valvular, other congenital cardiac defects include pulmonary stenosis, atrial septal defects and ventricular septal defects. It is associated with low birth weight and growth retardation in the first four years. They typically have a friendly personality, short attention span and anxiety.

17. ACDE

Psoriasis may affect any age but usually occurs over five years. Guttate psoriasis often follows a streptococcal or viral sore throat or ear infection. The nails are often involved, with distal nail separation from the nail bed (onycholysis), thickening and ridges, fine pitting is rare. 30% have a parent affected. Drugs such as beta-blockers and antimalarials can trigger the disease. May demonstrate Koebner's phenomenon, which is psoriasis along the sites of skin trauma, and Von Spitz sign, which is pinpoint bleeding on scratching a psoriatic plaque.

18. ABCD

Pityriasis rosea is associated with Human Herpes virus 7. It begins with a large herald patch on the trunk, upper arms, neck or thigh, and smaller lesions in a Christmas tree distribution, following the lines of the ribs posteriorly. No treatment is required but menthol in aqueous cream may help relieve any itch. It usually clears in 4 to 6 weeks.

19. BCDE

Epidermolysis bullosa is a group of genetically distinct disorders, in which the epidermis separates from the dermis. There is blister formation in response to mild friction or trauma. Severity of symptoms ranges from blistering on the hands and feet, to disabling and life-threatening forms. Treatment is symptomatic, there is no cure.

20. ACD

Erythrasma is caused by Corynebacterium minutissimum. It is usually seen as an orangey brown rash on flexural surfaces, and in the axilla or toe web spaces. The rash shows a coral pink fluorescence under Wood's light. It responds well to erythromycin or topical miconazole or fusidic acid.

21. ABCD

Koebner phenomenon is where skin lesions appear in the lines of trauma. It is seen in psoriasis, Lichen planus, molluscum contagiosum, viral warts and vitiligo. Some skin injuries can trigger the Koebner phenomenon, such as: insect bites, thermal burns, thumb sucking, BCG and influenza vaccinations, urticaria, phototherapy and immunosuppression.

22. ABCDE

Erythema multiforme is an immunologically mediated rash with target lesions, with a central papule, surrounded by an erythematous ring; it may be vesicular or bullous. It may be idiopathic but is usually precipitated by infection such as Mycoplasma, herpes simplex, HIV, Epstein Barr virus and lymphoma. It may be caused by drugs such as Sulphonamides and Penicillin. It is associated with connective tissue diseases such as; Systemic lupus erythematosus, Polyarteritis nodosa, Wegener's Granulomatosis and carcinomas.

23. BCDE

Hereditary angio-oedema is an autosomal dominant condition caused by a deficiency of C1 esterase inhibitor. There is swelling of the subcutaneous tissue. It may cause respiratory obstruction and can be life-threatening. It involves the lips, eyelids, genitalia, tongue or larynx.

24. All false

Infantile seborrhoeic dermatitis usually presents in the first two months of life with erythema and a scaling rash, affecting the face, neck, behind the ears, axilla, scalp, upper trunk, flexures and nappy area. Cause is unknown, maternal androgens have been implicated in infants. The child is unperturbed by it. It usually resolves spontaneously within a few weeks. It is associated with increased risk of developing atopic eczema, especially if there is a positive family history. Mild cases resolve with emollients, widespread body eruptions respond to topical corticosteroids.

25. ABCD

Haemangiomas present after birth anywhere on the body. They are commoner in females and preterm infants. Capillary haemangiomas may be associated with glaucoma if near the eye. Port wine stain is a developmental vascular malformation which is present at birth. It presents as a bright red or purple macule, usually on the face and neck, however it may be anywhere on the body. Capillary haemangiomas are associated with the Sturge-Weber syndrome, in which there is involvement of the ophthalmic division of the Trigeminal nerve. Large strawberry naevi are associated with high output cardiac failure from the shunting of large volumes of blood.

26. ABCD

The Sturge-Weber syndrome is a congenital condition which is associated with a capillary haemangioma or port wine stain in the distribution of the ophthalmic division of the Trigeminal nerve. It may present with intractable epilepsy in early infancy. There may be learning disability, hemiplegia, glaucoma and severe headaches.

27. ACDE

Patients with Mucopolysaccharidosis appear normal at birth, and usually present with developmental delay or regression. They may have hearing defects and eye defects such as squints, corneal clouding, retinal degeneration and glaucoma; hepatosplenomegaly, thoracic kyphosis and lumbar lordosis. It is associated with cardiac defects such as valvular lesions and cardiac failure.

28. BE

In mucopolysaccharidosis, development is usually normal up to 6 to 12 months of age, and then it slows down and regresses. There are course facies with thickened skull and frontal bossing. It is associated with umbilical and inguinal hernias. There is excretion of glycosaminoglycans in the urine. Treatment is with bone marrow transplantation, which significantly helps with the phenotype, however does not help with neurological features. The mainstay of treatment is supportive.

29. ACD

Hair loss is seen in hypothyroidism, hypopituitarism, homocystinuria, Acrodermatitis enteropathica and fungal infections such as tinea capitis, and in aplasia cutis. It can be caused by retinoids and heparin therapy.

30. CE

Candida infection of the nappy area includes the flexures. Irritant dermatitis occurs due to the irritant effect of urine on the skin, and may have a scalded skin appearance. Pityriasis rosea causes an itchy rash. Acrodermatitis enteropathica typically affects the mucocutaneous junctions, and the rash is seen mainly around the mouth and anus. It is due to a congenital defect in zinc transport.

31. BC

Down's syndrome affects one in 700 live births. It is associated with cardiovascular malformations in 40% particularly atrioventricular septal defects. Gastrointestinal abnormalities are seen in 6%, particularly duodenal atresia and Hirschsprung disease. Hearing loss is present in over 40% and is commonly due to middle ear disease. Haematological abnormalities particularly leukaemia is seen in one in 150. It is associated with cataracts in about 3%. Alzheimer's disease is seen in the majority by 40 years of age.

32. BCE

Accidental poisoning occurs most commonly in boys aged 1 to 4 years. There has been a marked reduction in the hospital admission rates for accidental poisoning, due to the introduction of child resistant containers. Intentional poisoning is usually seen in teenage girls. Activated charcoal is used to limit absorption of poison if ingested within one hour. Gastric lavage is only considered when a large quantity of toxic drug has been taken. Lead poisoning is seen in preschool children, and often results from pica. It is rare but potentially very serious, and is the commonest cause of chronic poisoning in children.

33. ABCE

Lead poisoning often results from pica, ingesting lead paint, lead pipes and leaded petrol. Children may present with failure to thrive, abdominal pain, vomiting, lead encephalopathy with behavioural disturbance, seizures, drowsiness or coma. Chronic exposure to lower levels may lead to mental retardation. There may be hypochromic anaemia with punctate basophilic stippling of neutrophils. X-rays of the knee or wrist may show lead lines, which appear as dense metaphyseal bands. Treatment involves removing the source, chelating agents such as D- penicillamine is given orally in mild cases, and intravenous Calcium Disodium Edetate (EDTA) in severe cases.

34. BD

Jaundice is prolonged if it lasts more than 14 days in term babies, and more than 21 days in preterm babies. Unconjugated hyperbilirubinaemia is commonly seen in physiological and breast milk jaundice, haemolysis and congenital hyperbilirubinaemia. Kernicterus results from high levels of lipid soluble unconjugated bilirubin crossing the blood brain barrier. Management is with phototherapy, hydration and treatment of the underlying cause. Conjugated hyperbilirubinaemia is most commonly due to neonatal hepatitis, biliary atresia, cystic fibrosis and alpha-1 trypsin deficiency. Surgery for biliary atresia should be performed within eight weeks. 80% will achieve bile drainage, after 8 weeks the success rate declines.

35. C

First-degree relatives of patients with coeliac disease have a 10% risk of developing the condition. It is associated with HLA DQ2 and DQ 8. Diagnosis is based on a combination of serological tests, small bowel biopsy and response to an exclusion diet. IgA tissue transglutaminase has a high sensitivity and specificity. IgA deficiency is common. Small bowel biopsy is done to confirm the diagnosis before starting a gluten-free diet. The characteristic features on biopsy are of subtotal villous atrophy, lymphocytosis and plasma cell infiltration of the lamina propria. This returns to normal on a gluten-free diet. A gluten-free diet is recommended for life.

36. BDE

Wilson's disease is an autosomal recessive disorder which leads to excessive deposition of copper in the liver and the nervous system, due to lack of caeruloplasmin. Signs and symptoms usually develop from the age of 10 years onwards and are rare under five years. Neurological abnormalities are common in the second decade and include slurred speech, choreoathetosis, tremors, dystonia and myoclonus. Other features include anaemia, jaundice, Kayser-Fleischer rings, hepatosplenomegaly, and change in personality and psychotic behaviour. It may be associated with Ricketts due to renal tubular dysfunction. There is low plasma concentration of caeruloplasmin and elevated 24-hour urinary copper excretion.

37. BCE

Alpha-1 antitrypsin deficiency is an autosomal recessive condition, and occurs in one in 2000 live births. It is the most common inherited cause of conjugated jaundice, and is associated with intrauterine growth retardation. Pulmonary disease is not significant in childhood, and may present in adults as emphysema. There may be intracranial haemorrhage from vitamin K deficiency, especially in breastfed infants. 50% of children presenting with neonatal hepatitis go on to develop chronic liver disease including, cirrhosis, portal hypertension and may require a liver transplant.

38. BDE

Alagilles's syndrome is a rare autosomal dominant condition which presents with prolonged jaundice and failure to thrive. There is conjugated hyperbilirubinaemia due to intrahepatic biliary hypoplasia. Characteristic facies, which develop later include; triangular facies, deep-set eyes, mild hypertelorism, and a small chin. There may be associated cardiac problems such as pulmonary stenosis, and renal tubular defects, skeletal abnormalities and eye defects. It is associated with delayed puberty and learning difficulties. Prognosis is variable with 50% of children surviving into adult life without a liver transplant.

39. ACE

Hepatitis B is a DNA virus. Vertical transmission of hepatitis B leads to a 70-90 per cent risk of transmission, whereas with hepatitis C it is rare, unless if there is co-infection with HIV. Symptomatic acute hepatitis B resolves completely in 90% of cases, and results in lifelong immunity, whereas at least 50% of acute hepatitis C infection leads to chronic hepatic infection. 15 to 30% of those with chronic hepatitis C infection progress to cirrhosis. Hepatitis D alone does not cause acute infectious hepatitis unless if it occurs as a super-infection with hepatitis B, in which case it progresses rapidly at all ages to chronic hepatitis, cirrhosis and hepatocellular carcinoma develops in 50-70% of cases.

40. CE

Autoimmune hepatitis occurs more commonly in girls. The mean age of presentation is 7 to 10 years. Diagnosis is based on hypergammaglobulinaemia with an IgG of more than 20 g/L or more than 1.5 times normal, and raised autoantibodies such as antinuclear antibody, anti- smooth muscle antibody and is associated with raised aminotransferases. Up to 90% of children respond to steroids and Azathioprine. There may be other autoimmune features, for example rash, arthritis, haemolytic anaemia or nephritis maybe present. Relapses are common and occur in 40% of cases.

41. ABC

Surfactant production is stimulated by steroids, prolactin, and thyroxine and beta agonists. It is inhibited by insulin. Surfactant is produced by Type II pneumocytes of the lung and is stimulated by alveolar distension. It is composed of phospholipids and proteins.

42. ABD

Surfactant administration reduces neonatal mortality by 30%. It reduces bronchopulmonary dysplasia and the incidence of pneumothorax; however it may cause pulmonary haemorrhage. It reduces intraventricular haemorrhage by over 40%. Surfactant reduces the risk of infection, and the need for admission to the neonatal intensive care unit.

43. ABE

Patent ductus arteriosus is a common condition in preterm babies. Small defects are generally asymptomatic, large defects may cause apnoea and bradycardia, poor growth and difficulty in feeding. Clinical features include: bounding pulse due to increased pulse pressure and systolic or continuous machinery murmur at the upper left sternal edge. Management is with fluid restriction and indomethacin. Surgery may be necessary if medical management fails.

44. ABCE

Cerebral haemorrhage occurs in 10 to 15% of infants born less than 32 weeks, most haemorrhages occur within the first 72 hours. Up to 50% are asymptomatic. And there is a more than 50% chance of being normal if the cranial scan is normal. Periventricular leukomalacia is seen in up to 10% of very low birth weight infants; there is a high risk of cerebral palsy with periventricular cysts. Intracranial lesions are more common following birth asphyxia and severe respiratory distress syndrome, and may progress to hydrocephalus and convulsions.

45. BC

Necrotising enterocolitis affects preterm infants in the first few weeks of life. It is caused by ischaemia of the bowel wall and infection, and is 6 to 10 times higher in those fed formula milk compared with those given breast milk. It presents with vomiting, blood in the stools and abdominal distension. Abdominal x-ray shows intestinal distension with thickening of the bowel wall and intramural air. Antenatal steroids are protective. Overall mortality is about 20%.

46. DE

Retinopathy of prematurity occurs due to arterial hyperoxia and retinal ischaemia, during retinal development before 32 weeks gestation. It occurs in 30 to 60% of very low birth weight infants. Screening is done and continued at six weeks postnatal age, and prognosis is good with stages 1 to 3 regressing spontaneously. Severe visual impairment occurs in about one per cent. Chronic lung disease of prematurity, also known as bronchopulmonary dysplasia; is defined as oxygen dependence at 28 days or at 36 weeks gestational age.

47. BCD

Kernicterus is caused by the deposition of unconjugated bilirubin in the basal ganglia and cerebellum. It presents with lethargy, hypotonia, poor feeding, high-pitched cry, opisthotonus position, seizures and coma. Spasticity usually resolves, but there may be sensorineural deafness, mental retardation and enamel dysplasia, which leads to permanent discolouration of the teeth.

48. BC

Diaphragmatic hernia occurs in one in 2500 births. It is more common on the left side. The main problem is due to associated pulmonary hypoplasia, and may lead to pneumothorax due to rigorous resuscitation. Chest x-ray shows bowel loops inside the thorax. With good treatment the mortality rate has decreased from 50 to 60%, to 20 to 40%.

49. ABCDE

Neonatal sepsis may present with fever or hypothermia; hyperglycaemia or hypoglycaemia may be a feature. There is usually poor perfusion and evidence of shock and coagulopathy, with petechia, purpura and neutropenia. Opisthotonus posture may be seen in meningitis. Meconium staining of the liquor at birth is seen in Listeria monocytogenes infection.

50. CE

Cleft lip and palate is diagnosed antenatally on ultrasound scan. The incidence is one in 1000. Cleft lip is repaired at approximately 2 to 3 months of age and the palate is repaired at 6 months to a year. Infants are prone to otitis media. Adenoidectomy is best avoided, as the resultant gap between the abnormal palate and nasopharynx will exacerbate feeding problems and the nasal quality of speech.

51. ABDE

Pierre-Robin sequence is characterised by three features: Micrognathia, glossoptosis and cleft palate. It is associated with congenital heart disease, and may result in cyanotic episodes due to obstruction to the upper airways from the large tongue particularly during sleep.

Prone positioning may help, allowing the tongue to fall forward, but occasionally tracheostomy may be required. The baby is at risk of failure to thrive in the first few months due to feeding difficulties, then as the mandible grows, the problems resolve. Cleft palate is generally repaired between 9 and 18 months of age. Airway problems improve with growth.

52. E

Gastroschisis is rarely associated with other malformations except for intestinal atresia in 10%, whereas Exomphalos is associated with chromosomal defects including trisomy 13, 18 and 21, and other malformations in 40 to 70% of cases. In Gastroschisis, the bowel is eviscerated and not covered by a sac, whereas in exomphalos, the hernia protrudes through a defect into the base of the umbilical cord and is therefore covered by a sac of amnion. Gastroschisis requires surgical closure as soon as possible, whereas exomphalos is closed in one or more stages.

53. BCE

85% of oesophageal atresias occur with a tracheo-oesophageal fistula. Tracheo -oesophageal fistula presents with persistent salivation and choking due to aspiration after feeding. Hirschsprung disease usually presents in infancy with poor feeding, abdominal distension, vomiting and delayed passage of meconium. It may present with enterocolitis in 15%. In small bowel obstruction there is persistent vomiting which is bile-stained if the obstruction is below the ampulla of Vater.

54. BD

Beckwith- Wiedemann syndrome is associated with fetal overgrowth, and is due to defects on chromosome 11. It presents with macrosomia, organomegaly, macroglossia and hemi-hypertrophy. There may be associated congenital anomalies, with exomphalos in 50% of cases. Hypoglycaemia occurs due to islet cell hyperplasia. It is associated with malignancy in 5%, more so in children with hemi- hypertrophy; most commonly with Wilm's tumour, then hepatoblastoma and Neuroblastoma.

55. BCE

Acute lymphoblastic leukaemia is the most common malignancy in childhood, followed by brain tumours and lymphomas. Childhood cancer is more common in boys. Neuroblastoma and Wilm's tumour usually present in the first five years of life. According to data from the Office for National Statistics, cancer is the second leading cause of death in children after accidents.

56. E

Acute lymphoblastic leukaemia (ALL) accounts for 80% of leukaemia in children. Poor prognostic signs in ALL include; white cell count less than 50 x 10 9/l, age less than 2 and over 10 years, male sex, Philadelphia chromosome, Afro-Caribbean ethnicity and central nervous system disease. The five-year survival rate is 80%.

57. DE

Hodgkin's disease rarely occurs before the age of five years. It usually presents with painless cervical lymphadenopathy. B- symptoms such as fever and night sweats, weight loss and pruritus are common in advanced stages. Reed -Sternberg cells are pathognomonic of Hodgkin's lymphoma. Non-Hodgkin's lymphoma originates from either the B or T lymphocytes. The abdomen is usually affected with B-cell disease, it may present as an intussusception. T -cell Non-Hodgkin's lymphoma, typically presents with a mass in the mediastinum. B cell lymphomas account for 85% of all Non –Hodgkin's lymphomas.

58. ACD

Neuroblastoma is a tumour of the autonomic nervous system, arising from crest tissue in the adrenal medulla and sympathetic chain. It is most commonly seen up to 2 years of age. Spontaneous regression may occur, or it may behave as an aggressive tumour with widespread metastasis. Poor prognosis is seen in children over 18 months, and in those with the N- myc oncogene. Urinary and plasma vanillylmandelic acid and homovanillic acid may be raised.

59. AC

Wilm's tumour or nephroblastoma is a tumour of the developing kidney. The child is usually well. Signs include: painless abdominal mass in up to 80%, haematuria in about 20% and hypertension may occur in some children. 80% present before five years of age. It is associated with aniridia, and Beckwith- Wiedemann syndrome. Prognosis is very good with more than 90% 5 year survival rate.

60. BCDE

Nephrotic syndrome comprises of a triad of proteinuria, oedema and hypoalbuminaemia. It is twice as common in boys. 85% of cases are due to minimal change disease, other causes include focal segmental glomerulosclerosis and membranous glomerulonephritis. It is often precipitated by respiratory infections, malaria, vasculitis and allergens.

Answers Paper 3

The following statements are true.

1. ACDE

Osteosarcoma is twice as common as Ewing's sarcoma and is seen in the metaphyses of long bones. They are uncommon before puberty and peak in teenage. Usually present with localised bone pain, lung metastasis is common. Ewing's sarcoma presents in the axial skeleton i.e. in the pelvis, ribs and vertebrae.

2. ABCE

Retinoblastoma is the most common intraocular malignancy in childhood. 90% present within the first three years of life. It maybe familial in 25% of cases, and may be associated with mutations on chromosome 13. It presents with visual deterioration, squint, absent light reflex or leukocoria is seen in 60%. There is a significant risk of a second malignancy, most commonly osteosarcoma.

3. BD

Prune-belly syndrome or megacystis- mega ureter is commoner in males, usually sporadic with a 1% recurrence risk in siblings. There is deficient abdominal wall musculature, with skin hanging in wrinkled folds and distended abdomen. Kidneys may be palpable due to hydronephrosis and large neurogenic bladder. It is associated with congenital dislocation of the hips and talipes, cryptorchidism and pulmonary hypoplasia.

4. BCDE

Up to 3% of girls and 1% of boys suffer from urinary tract infection (UTI) during childhood. Proteus infection is more common in boys, as it may be present under the prepuce. It predisposes to the formation of phosphate stones .Pseudomonas infection is an indicator of structural abnormality in the urinary tract .UTIs may present with vomiting, diarrhoea, poor feeding and prolonged neonatal jaundice in infancy.

5. ABCDE

Henoch- Schonlein purpura is an inflammation of the small vessels, associated with IgA immune complexes. It is often precipitated by an upper respiratory tract infection, particularly due to haemolytic streptococci. It is more common in males, and generally presents after three years of age. Clinical features include arthritis, colicky abdominal pain and a palpable, purpuric rash, usually seen on the feet, legs and buttocks, and cutaneous nodules over the elbows and knees. Follow-up is necessary as hypertension and declining renal function may develop after an interval of several years.

6. CDE

Horner's syndrome involves ptosis, miosis, enophthalmos, and ipsilateral anhidrosis. The direct and consensual light reflexes are normal. In congenital cases there is heterochromia of the irides. It may be caused by brachial plexus damage at birth, leading to sympathetic denervation of the eye; surgery or tumours such as neuroblastoma, or tumours in the mediastinum or cervical region.

7. ABCDE

In constitutional obesity, puberty is advanced so the final height centile is less than in childhood, and the height is usually appropriate or may be tall for their parent's height. Androgen excess may lead to tall stature. The child is tall and long-legged in homocystinuria. Soto's syndrome is associated with a large head and characteristic facial features, excessive linear growth during the first few years and learning disability.

8. BD

Cerebral palsy is a non-progressive lesion, caused by injury to the motor pathways in the developing brain, leading to a chronic disorder of movement. There may be developmental delay, learning difficulties are present in around 60% .It is associated with epilepsy, visual impairment in 20% ,hearing loss, speech and language delay and behavioural disorders.

9. BCE

In whooping cough, whoop is often absent in infants. Vomiting may occur after paroxysms of coughing and apnoea may follow in babies. Erythromycin reduces infectivity but has minimal effect on the course of the disease unless if given in the first week of the illness. Salbutamol, steroids and antitussives have no proven role in whooping cough. It is a notifiable disease.

10. BE

In ataxic cerebral palsy there are symmetric, uncoordinated movements. Signs are usually symmetrical with early hypotonia, poor balance and delayed motor development, later uncoordinated moments and intention tremor, reflecting dysfunction in the cerebellum or its pathways occurs. Cerebral development occurs normally, 50% have some form of learning disability. Abnormal movements are seen in over one year of age in the dyskinetic group.

11. C

Ataxia telangiectasia is a multisystem disease with autosomal recessive inheritance. Telangiectasias are present from about two years of age, and are seen in the conjunctiva, neck and shoulders. Clinical features include; recurrent infections due to immunodeficiency, with lymphopenia and hypogammaglobulinaemia, progressive neurological impairment, cerebellar ataxia, global developmental delay and increased risk of lympho- reticular malignancy especially acute lymphoblastic leukaemia. Many are wheelchair bound in early adolescence.

12. BDE

Friedreich's ataxia is an autosomal recessive condition, which presents with progressive clumsiness due to a lower motor lesion with wasting and absent deep tendon reflexes, more in the legs, and impaired joint position and vibration sense. It is associated with diabetes mellitus in 10 to 25% of cases.

13. ADE

A long PR interval is seen in Duchenne's muscular dystrophy, hypothermia and Ebstein's anomaly and diphtheria.

14. ABCE

Non-accidental injury to the head in children involves skull fractures, especially depressed fractures, occipital fractures, or those crossing the suture lines involving two bones. Subdural haematoma is seen almost exclusively in non-accidental injury in infants or toddlers, and is usually caused by shaking. Lumbar puncture should be avoided as the haemorrhage may extend. There may be associated retinal haemorrhages. Extradural haemorrhages are usually associated with skull fractures and may present in young children with anaemia and shock.

15. DE

All babies born to Hepatitis B infected mothers should receive hepatitis B immunoglobulin. According to the World Health Organisation (WHO 1996) there is no evidence that breastfeeding increases the mother to child transmission of Hepatitis B in immunised infants. Untreated active tuberculosis is a contraindication to breastfeeding. The baby is immunised at birth, and treated with a course of isoniazid.

16. CD

The long-term management of diabetes in children as per NICE Guidance (August 2015), should be carried out by a multi-disciplinary team. The target HbA1C should be less than 7.5%, with an ideal target of 48 mmol/l or 6.5%, to reduce the risk of long-term complications, as well as hypoglycaemia. Screening should be arranged with annual blood pressure checks, microalbuminuria and retinopathy from 12 years of age. Coeliac disease should be screened for at diagnosis; however Coeliac UK recommends screening every 3 years till 18. Thyroid disease should be screened for at diagnosis and annually.

17. ABCE

Guillain- Barre syndrome may occur at any age, but in childhood it peaks at 4-7 years. It typically presents 2-3 weeks after a viral infection, and classically after Campylobacter enteritis. There is demyelination of the peripheral nerves leading to a progressive weakness, usually affecting the lower limbs. The autonomic nervous system may be involved with sweating, orthostatic hypotension, hypertension and tachyarrhythmia. The cerebral spinal fluid (CSF) white cell count is not raised; there is a high CSF protein. Cranial nerves may be involved, the facial nerve is involved in 50%, and dysphagia due to ninth and 10th nerve involvement is also seen.

18. BCE

In Guillain- Barre syndrome there is sudden onset of weakness which usually affects the lower limbs symmetrically, with ascending paralysis and pain.

Treatment is supportive; steroids do not help, and may delay recovery. Ventilation may be needed as respiratory paralysis occurs in up to 20% of untreated cases. Immunoglobulins and plasmapheresis may be needed. Most children recover within a few weeks to months, and 95% recover within two years. Mortality rate is 2 to 3% in children, and 5-10 % may have a permanent deficit.

19. ABE

Bell's palsy is usually idiopathic but can be of viral aetiology. In an upper motor neuron lesion there is sparing of the forehead, the paralysis is usually unilateral. A full systemic and neurological examination should be done, as it may be associated with coarctation of the aorta, and can cause hypertension. Conjunctivitis may occur due to incomplete closure of the eye, and will require a patch to close the eye. Acyclovir is used; the evidence for use of steroids in children is limited. Most children recover fully, but can take a few months in some cases.

20. ABE

Juvenile myasthenia gravis is an autoimmune disorder; with antibodies against the acetylcholine receptor. It usually presents after 10 years of age, with muscle weakness which increases with exertion, ptosis, loss of facial expression and difficulty in chewing. Treatment options include, anti-cholinesterase, steroids, plasma exchange for crises, and thymectomy may be needed if a thymoma is present.

21. ACE

There are two forms of neurofibromatosis; type I or Von Recklinghausen's disease is coded on chromosome 17 and Type II on chromosome 22, but up to 50% are due to new mutations and may be autosomal dominant. There may be short stature, type I is associated with mental retardation and epilepsy. Renal artery stenosis and hypertension are known complications.

22. AC

Skin involvement in tuberous sclerosis includes, ash-leaf macules, shagreen patches, especially over the lumbosacral area and adenoma sebaceum on the face. Cafe au-lait patches are present in 5% of cases. Nail involvement includes subungual fibromas which are rare in childhood. There may be gingival fibromas in the mouth. Mental retardation is seen in 50%, and includes developmental delay and learning difficulties. Tuberous sclerosis is associated with cardiac rhabdomyomata which are detectable antenatally, and are usually asymptomatic with no signs and resolve spontaneously during childhood.

23. ABCE

Mucopolysaccharidosis is a group of progressive multisystem disorders, characterised by coarse facial features, thickened skin, thoracic kyphosis, lumbar lordosis and hepatosplenomegaly. There may be normal growth and development up to 6 to 12 months of age, followed by developmental delay and loss of skills. It is associated with corneal clouding, retinal degeneration, glaucoma and conductive deafness. Valvular heart lesions may lead to cardiac failure.

24. AE

Dermatomyositis comprises of muscle pain and weakness, characteristic skin rash and vasculitis. It is more common in girls and peaks at 4 to 10 years of age. There is a periorbital skin rash on the face, and erythematous rash is seen on the extensor surfaces of joints. There is an insidious onset of progressive muscle weakness over several weeks with post-exercise pain in the majority of cases. ESR is usually normal but creatinine kinase and lactate dehydrogenase are elevated.

25. CD

Myotonic dystrophy is an autosomal dominant condition, with expansion of trinucleotide repeats on chromosome 19. It presents with severe hypotonia at birth and feeding difficulties. It leads to progressive weakness. There is cardiac involvement with cardiomyopathy, arrhythmias and mitral valve prolapse. It is associated with diabetes mellitus and mental retardation.

26. CDE

Infectious mononucleosis or Glandular fever is caused by the Epstein-Barr virus which affects the pharynx and the B lymphocytes. Maculopapular rash is seen in 5-15%. An itchy morbilliform rash may appear in 30 to 70% and in some studies up to 90% of cases, 7 to 10 days after treatment with beta lactam antibiotics like amoxicillin, ampicillin or a cephalosporin. It is a hypersensitivity to the antibiotic when infected with the virus, but does not occur when the antibiotics are taken again. Jaundice may be a feature and there is hepatomegaly in 30%, and splenomegaly in 50%. Diagnosis is supported by the presence of atypical lymphocytes and heterophil antibodies, Paul-Bunnell or Monospot test, which may be negative in young children and serological testing.

27. CE

Human herpes virus 6 causes Roseola infantum, and is a common cause of febrile convulsions. There is high fever and malaise, lasting a few days, followed by a generalised macular rash. The human herpes virus 8 usually does not affect normal healthy children, and causes Kaposi's sarcoma in immunocompromised children. Herpes simplex virus 2 infection is seen in sexually active adolescents, and is rare in younger children. Aseptic meningitis due to herpes simplex virus usually resolves without sequelae, however encephalitis is a very serious condition with a mortality rate of up to 70% if untreated. Herpes simplex virus infection involving the eye causes blepharitis, conjunctivitis, and may involve the cornea producing dendritic ulcers which can lead to loss of vision.

28. CD

Mumps is spread by respiratory droplets. The incubation period is 14 to 21 days. Plasma amylase is often elevated due to pancreatic involvement. It may lead to sensorineural hearing loss which is usually unilateral. Transient orchitis is rare in childhood, but is seen in 15 to 35% in adolescents and is usually unilateral. Parotid gland swelling may or may not be present. Mumps is a notifiable disease.

29. ABE

Pox virus causes Molluscum contagiosum, and is spread by direct contact. Human papilloma virus causes warts, and is spread by direct contact. Coxsackie virus is an Enterovirus, and is usually spread by the faecal- oral route, however occasionally it is spread by droplets. It causes hand –foot and mouth disease.

30. CD

Macrocephaly is defined as occipitofrontal head circumference over 2.5 standard deviations for age sex and gestational age. It may be familial, and is seen in hydrocephalus, achondroplasia, neurofibromatosis, tuberous sclerosis, Soto's syndrome and metabolic conditions such as mucopolysaccharidosis.

31. CD

Meningococcal meningitis is the most common cause of community-acquired bacterial meningitis in the UK. It generally resolves without any long-term neurological sequelae. Pneumococcal meningitis is associated with higher risk of morbidity, with 30% of survivors having neurological impairment; mortality can be up to 10%. Tuberculous meningitis is rare but serious, and affects children of all ages. In children it presents with non-specific symptoms of low grade fever, aches, reduced appetite and tiredness for 2 to 8 weeks. After which there may be symptoms of meningitis; like severe headache, vomiting, neck stiffness, photophobia and seizures. Rifampicin is given as prophylaxis against meningococcal meningitis to all household contacts.

32. CD

Childhood tics affect around 25% of children and are more common in boys and usually start at the age of seven years. There may be a positive family history, they may worsen with anxiety. They can be voluntarily suppressed to some extent, and are worse when the child is inactive for example watching TV, and usually disappear when actively concentrating. Tics usually resolve spontaneously, however treatment with haloperidol or clonidine may be needed. Tourette's syndrome is a chronic disorder which includes multiple motor and vocal tics.

33. CD

Diabetes affects around 2 in 10,000 children. There is an increased risk in those who have HLA DR 3 and 4. Peak age at presentation is at 4 to 6 years and 10 to 14 years. As per NICE Guidance (August 2015), diabetes in children should be confirmed by a random plasma glucose of 11 mmols/l in the presence of classical symptoms, such as polyuria, polydipsia, weight loss or tiredness, or by a raised HbA1C. It is associated with Down's syndrome and Prader Willi syndrome.

34. ABD

Inborn errors of metabolism usually present in the neonatal period with persistent or recurrent vomiting, poor feeding and failure to thrive. Phenylketonuria presents with developmental delay at 6 to 12 months, learning disability and behavioural problems. Homocysteinuria is associated with tall stature, developmental delay and downward subluxation of the lens. There may be pendular nystagmus and photophobia in albinism. Galactosaemia presents with hypoglycaemia due to the inability to mobilise glucose from galactose. When lactose –containing milk feeds e.g. Breast or infant formula are introduced, affected infants eat poorly, vomit and develop jaundice, hepatomegaly and hepatic failure.

35. ABE

Sickle cell disease is associated with delayed puberty and short stature. Other long-term problems include cardiomegaly and heart failure, renal dysfunction, gall stones and leg ulcers. Adenotonsillar hypertrophy may lead to vaso- occlusive crises and sleep apnoea syndrome. Vaso- occlusive crises will be prevented if the proportion of HbS is less than 30%. Exchange transfusion is indicated for priapism and cerebral and pulmonary infarction.

36. ABCDE

Complications of obesity include insulin resistance and Type II diabetes, obstructive sleep apnoea and heart failure, psychological problems, fatty liver and slipped upper femoral epiphyses, with tibia vara or bow legs.

37. ABCE

Intrauterine growth retardation and extreme prematurity can result in short stature. Psychosocial or emotional deprivation may also result in short stature.

Constitutional obesity leads to tall stature. Average growth during puberty is 30 cm.

38. E

Puberty starts on average at 10 years in girls; the first sign is breast development, followed by pubic and axillary hair. Menarche occurs 2.5 years after the onset of puberty and signals the end of growth. Puberty in boys starts on average at 12 years, the first sign is testicular enlargement to 4ml, followed by pubic hair and penile growth. The height spurt in boys occurs with testicular volumes of 10-12 ml. Bone age measurement is usually done from an x-ray of the hand and wrist.

39. ACD

Precocious puberty is almost always pathological in males, whereas no underlying cause is usually found in girls. True precocious puberty is due to premature pulsatile activity of GnRH, which may be idiopathic, familial or due to central nervous system tumours. Craniopharyngioma causes delayed puberty. Gonadotropin independent precocious puberty is seen in ovarian and testicular tumours, and liver or adrenal tumours.

40. BDE

Congenital adrenal hyperplasia is an autosomal recessive condition, in which there is deficiency of the 21 hydroxylase enzyme, which leads to a block in the production of cortisol and aldosterone, with resulting increased levels of 17 hydroxyprogesterone in the blood. It presents with ambiguous genitalia in girls, and precocious puberty in boys. There is metabolic acidosis, hypoglycaemia, salt losing crisis and hypotension.

41. ABDE

Irritable hip is the most common cause of acute hip pain in children. It is a benign inflammation of the hip joint and is usually idiopathic but may follow a viral infection. There is reduced range of movement with pain. The main differential diagnosis is septic arthritis in which there is pain at rest, tenderness, fever and raised C reactive protein. Management is with analgesics and physiotherapy. It usually improves within a few days.

42. ABCDE

Osteogenesis imperfecta is due to a defect in type one collagen. It may be autosomal dominant or recessive. It is associated with increased fragility of bones, fractures maybe present before birth, short stature, blue sclera, conductive hearing loss, ligamentous laxity and scoliosis. The aim of management is to reduce the risk and aid in fracture management and rehabilitation.

43. C

Perthes disease occurs most commonly at 5 to 10 years of age. It is more common in boys with a male to female ratio of 4:1. It is bilateral in 10 to 20% of cases. There is insidious onset of hip pain, reduced movement and limping and there may be referred pain to the knee. Investigation is by x-ray or MRI scans. Prognosis is good under six years of age and with less than half of the epiphysis involved. In children over six years there is increased chance of deformity and degenerative arthritis. Management is with bed rest and maintaining the hip in abduction, however femoral or pelvic osteotomy may be needed.

44. C

Slipped upper femoral epiphysis is due to the displacement of the epiphyses of the femoral head posterio- inferiorly. It is commonly seen in boys aged 10 to 15 years. Presentation is with a limp or hip pain referred to the knee. The leg is shortened and externally rotated. It is bilateral in 25% of cases, and obesity is a risk factor. There is increased incidence in family members. Treatment is usually surgical fixation of the epiphyses.

45. BCE

Slipped upper femoral epiphyses may occur in association with endocrine problems such as hypothyroidism, Pseudo hypopituitarism, obesity, and precocious puberty and growth hormone disorders.

46. BE

Talipes equinovarus, also called clubfoot, has an incidence of 1 in 1000 .It is commoner in males, with a male to female ratio of 2:1. It may run in families and is associated with developmental dysplasia of the hip and spina bifida. The foot is inverted and supinated; the forefoot is adducted. The heel is rotated inwards and in planter flexion. The affected foot is shorter and the calf muscles are thinner. The position is fixed. Treatment may be non-surgical with serial casting and splinting. Corrective surgery is usually performed at 6 to 12 months of age.

47. CDE

Wilson disease and infantile polycystic renal failure are autosomal recessive conditions, whereas Peutz-Jegher's disease, adult polycystic kidney disease and hereditary spherocytosis are autosomal dominant.

48. ACDE

Cytomegalovirus retinitis leads to increased incidence of cataract. Rubella and Toxoplasma also cause cataracts. Rubella causes congenital heart defects.

49. C

A baby normally transfers objects at 6 months. Mouthing is seen at 6 months. A 2-year-old child can build a tower of 8 bricks. A 3-year-old child can copy a circle and a 5-year-old can copy a triangle.

50. E

Protein C deficiency is an autosomal dominant condition due to a defect on chromosome 2. Von Willebrand's disease is an autosomal dominant condition with a defect on chromosome 12. Gilbert's disease and hyperlipidaemia are autosomal dominant conditions. Alpha-1 antitrypsin deficiency is an autosomal recessive condition with a defect on chromosome 14.

51. AD

Duchenne muscular dystrophy and glucose 6-phosphate dehydrogenase deficiency are X-linked recessive diseases. Myotonic dystrophy is autosomal dominant. Galactosaemia and haemochromatosis are autosomal recessive.

52. BC

There are two HPV vaccines available in the UK; Cevarix and Gardasil. Cevarix is a bivalent vaccine protecting against HPV 16 and 18. Gardasil is a quadrivalent vaccine, protecting against four strains of HPV; HPV 16, 18, 6 and 11. It protects against genital warts as well as cervical cancer. From September 2008, HPV vaccination is routinely recommended for girls at 12 to 13 years of age. The UK HPV immunisation programme switched from Cevarix to Gardasil from September 2012. Both vaccines are over 99% effective at preventing precancerous lesions associated with HPV 16 or 18 in young women. Gardasil is licensed from nine years, however vaccination is not routinely recommended for 9 to 12 year old girls. If the course is interrupted, it should be resumed, allowing the appropriate interval between subsequent doses. The vaccination schedule is 0, 1 and six months, and should be given within a 12 month period. Patients with HIV infection should be considered for HPV vaccination.

53. CDE

Sudden infant death syndrome (SIDS) is the sudden unexplained death of an infant less than one year of age. Incidence has reduced in the UK since the introduction of the back to sleep campaign. It occurs most commonly at 2 to 4 months with a peak at 12 weeks. It is associated with the baby sleeping prone, overheating with too many clothes or covers, low income parents, overcrowded housing, single unsupported mothers, bed-sharing with parents, maternal smoking during pregnancy and after. However, sharing the parent's room but not the bed reduces the risk of SIDS. It is more common in boys and multiple birth, low-birth-weight babies and preterm delivery. Mothers aged less than 20 years have three times the risk of mothers aged 25 to 29 years.

54. C

In the UK about 50% of Afro-Caribbean children live in a single parent household.15% of white and less than 10% of Asian children live in single-parent households. According to the Office of National Statistics 2014, (data released March 2016), the under 18 conception rate for England and Wales was 22.9 per 1000 females aged 15 to 17 years, which is the lowest since 1969. According to the Department of Health 2009, most children have had alcohol by the age of 15 years. Since 1990 the amount of alcohol consumed by 11 to 15 year olds has doubled. According to the government's NHS information centre 2014, 35% of 15 year olds had ever smoked, and 30% of 15 year olds had personal experience of using drugs. Girls are more likely to be regular smokers than boys. Upto 15% of children smoke regularly. 40% of adult smokers started at less than 16 years of age.

55. ADE

Rota virus and Hepatitis C are RNA viruses, as are Influenza, measles, mumps, rubella, respiratory syncytial virus and rabies. Whereas hepatitis B, herpes simplex, varicella zoster, papilloma virus and molluscum contagiosum are DNA viruses.

56. ACE

Atrial septal defect causes a left to right shunt. 80% are due to a secundum defect. It may present with recurrent chest infections and wheeze. It is usually asymptomatic with a soft systolic murmur at the upper left sternal edge and a fixed split S2. Arrhythmias may occur in the fourth decade onwards and are usually atrial fibrillation. Atrial septal defect is seen in fetal alcohol syndrome, Down's syndrome and Noonan's syndrome. Chest x-ray shows increased pulmonary vascular markings. There is partial right bundle branch block and right ventricular hypertrophy on ECG. Closure is done at 3 to 5 years.

57. DE

Ventricular septal defects are seen in trisomy 18 and 21. Small defects are asymptomatic in 80% of cases, whereas a large defect leads to heart failure which may be symptomatic in the first few weeks of life. Small defects are associated with loud murmurs. Chest x-ray shows increased pulmonary vascular markings and cardiomegaly in large defects. Small defects usually close spontaneously, but large defects require surgical closure at 3 to 5 months.

58. BCDE

Most children with pulmonary stenosis are asymptomatic. There is an ejection systolic murmur at the upper sternal edge. It may be caused by the maternal ingestion of Phenytoin and Valproate antenatally. It is associated with Noonan syndrome, William's syndrome and Trisomy 18. The ECG shows right ventricular hypertrophy. Antibiotic prophylaxis is required.

59. ABD

Mild aortic stenosis is usually asymptomatic, however severe defects may present in the neonate, with heart failure and collapse. In childhood there may be reduced exercise tolerance, chest pain or syncope. The child is usually well grown. It is commoner in boys and is a feature of William's syndrome and Turner's syndrome. There is an ejection systolic murmur at the upper sternal edge. Chest x ray shows prominent left ventricle and post-stenotic dilatation of the ascending aorta. ECG shows left ventricular hypertrophy. Treatment is with balloon or surgical valvotomy.

60. ABC

Tetralogy of Fallot comprises of ventricular septal defect, pulmonary stenosis, over-riding aorta and right ventricular hypertrophy, leading to a right to left shunt. It may present with severe cyanosis at birth with a loud murmur at the upper sternal edge. The child may present with inconsolable crying, irritability and cyanosis, known as a "Tet spell "and is due to severe hypoxia and breathlessness. Chest x-ray is usually normal but there may be a boot- shaped heart with right ventricular hypertrophy and an upper tilted apex and oligaemic lung fields.

Answers Paper 4

The following statements are true.

1. CDE

Tetralogy of Fallot is usually asymptomatic. The volume work of the heart is less than normal; therefore heart failure does not occur. The systolic murmur softens or disappears during a Tet spell and returns when the spell is over. Thromboembolic stroke associated with polycythaemia due to persistent hypoxia may occur. Cerebral abscess is a known complication.

2. BE

A child can sit briefly or with support at six months, and unsupported at nine months. A 12 month old child can say two words with meaning; the limit age is 18 months. For 2 or 3 word sentences the limit age is 30 months.

3. ABCD

Sleep apnoea may lead to failure to thrive and developmental delay, daytime somnolence and pulmonary hypertension. Adeno- tonsillectomy is usually curative.

4. CDE

The cystic fibrosis gene is located on chromosome 7, with a carrier frequency of 1:25, causing disease in 1:2500 births of white babies. It presents with frequent chest infections, failure to thrive and prolonged jaundice in infancy. Pancreatic exocrine insufficiency presents with steatorrhoea and faltering growth, nutritional supplements and fat-soluble vitamins are required. It is associated with nasal polyps in 30% of cases. Diabetes is commoner in older children, along with cirrhosis, distal intestinal obstruction, rectal prolapse, pneumothorax, sterility in males and psychological problems.

5. CDE

Asthma affects 10 to 15% of school children, and causes 15 to 20 deaths in children per year in the UK. The main symptom in the preschool child is nocturnal cough.

6. ACDE

Abdominal pain is a very common symptom in childhood. Mesenteric adenitis is a common cause of abdominal pain in children especially after an upper respiratory tract infection. Malrotation may present with dark green bilious vomiting in the first few days of life, and needs urgent investigation. Meckel's diverticulum may present with severe rectal bleeding, and as intussusception. In which case there may be acute abdominal pain and shock.

7. BDE

Recurrent abdominal pain is defined as three or more episodes of abdominal pain severe enough to prevent activities, occurring over a period of three months. It is seen in 10 to 15% of children aged 5 to 15 years. In 90% of cases, no organic cause is found. The pain is characteristically around the umbilicus. Examination and investigations are usually normal. 50% improve spontaneously, in 25% the symptoms take some months to resolve, and the remaining 25% may have symptoms which persist till adulthood. Recurrent abdominal pain may be attributed to irritable bowel syndrome, non-ulcer dyspepsia and abdominal migraine.

8. BD

The frequency of coeliac disease is decreasing in the UK. It usually presents at 6 to 18 months of life, any time after gluten is introduced in the diet. Prevalence is 1%. It is associated with HLA DQ 2 and 8; there is an increased incidence in first-degree relatives. IgA tissue transglutaminase has 95 to 97% sensitivity for coeliac disease and a specificity of 98 to 100%. There is increased risk in patients with IgA deficiency. The only effective treatment is a gluten-free diet for life, which can reduce the risk of intestinal lymphoma in adulthood.

9. BCD

Raised sweat sodium or a false positive sweat test, is seen in: hypothyroidism, glucose 6 phosphate dehydrogenase deficiency, nephrotic syndrome, adrenal insufficiency, diabetes insipidus and severe malnutrition.

10. ABDE

Lyme disease is caused by the spirochaete, Borrelia burgdorferi, which is transmitted by a tick bite. It causes erythema migrans, which starts as a rash from the site of the tick bite, as a painless red expanding lesion to a large annular lesion, along with fever malaise and headache. It may lead to cranial nerve palsies especially affecting the seventh nerve and meningitis. There may be cardiac involvement with myocarditis which can lead to heart block. Arthralgia occurs in up to 50%, and varies from brief migratory arthralgia, to acute asymmetric mono and oligo arthritis of the large joints. Diagnosis is by serological testing, and the drug of choice in children over 12 years is doxycycline, and amoxicillin in younger children.

11. E

Kawasaki's disease is a systemic vasculitis affecting small and medium-sized arteries. It occurs in children aged between six months to 5 years, with peak incidence at 9 to 11 months. It is most common in Japanese children. The cause is unknown. The coronary arteries are affected in one third of cases and are best seen on echocardiogram. It may lead to myocardial ischaemia and sudden death. Treatment is with intravenous immunoglobulin and aspirin.

12. ABE

Setting speed limits is an example of primary prevention. Teaching parents first aid skills, is a type of tertiary prevention.

13. ACD

Seat belts and smoke alarms are examples of secondary prevention. Genetic counselling and immunisations are aimed at primary prevention.

14. CDE

Sickle cell disease usually presents after six months when haemoglobin F switches to haemoglobin A. Although the anaemia maybe severe, symptoms are usually mild. Neurological complications include cognitive defects due to silent brain infarcts and stroke. Penicillin prophylaxis and pneumococcal vaccination is recommended.

15. ADE

Pyloric stenosis occurs in 1 in 500 to 1000 live births, with a male to female ratio of 4:1. There may be a positive family history. 30-40% of cases occur in first-born children. It is more commonly seen in Caucasians of northern European descent, less so in African/Americans and is rare in Asians. There is hypokalaemia from persistent vomiting with hypochloraemic metabolic alkalosis. Unconjugated hyperbilirubinaemia may be present.

16. ABD

Kallmann's syndrome is a genetic disorder with hypogonadotrophic hypogonadism, causing delayed puberty with absent secondary sexual characteristics, mild to moderate mental retardation, renal agenesis and anosmia. There is a positive response to gonadotropin releasing hormone stimulation. 47XXY is Klinefelter's syndrome.

17. ACE

Causes of a prolonged QT on ECG are: hypocalcaemia, hypomagnesaemia, hypokalaemia, hypothermia, head injury and drugs such as erythromycin and domperidone.

18. ACD

Jaundice is seen in 30 to 40% of normal term babies. It is commoner in exclusively breast-fed babies. Unconjugated hyperbilirubinaemia is seen in physiological jaundice in the first few weeks of life, which is treated with phototherapy. Alpha-1 antitrypsin deficiency causes conjugated hyperbilirubinaemia.

19. AD

Absence of the red reflex is seen in retinoblastoma. The rooting reflex disappears at around four months of age. The palmar grasp reflex persists till three months, and for the foot, till 7 to 8 months of age. The stepping reflex disappears at two months.

20. BDE

Sudden infant death syndrome has an incidence of 0.4 per 1000 live births in the UK. It is commoner in infants aged 4 to 16 weeks, males, sleeping in the prone position, and bed- sharing with parents. It is associated with social deprivation, maternal smoking, low-birth-weight and prematurity. The use of a pacifier or dummy may be protective, as it may prevent the baby from sleeping deeply.

21. BC

The incubation period of chicken pox is 11 to 24 days. An infected child should be excluded from school until the rash crusts over. Aciclovir is not normally recommended in healthy children; however it can be given if the presentation is within 24 hours of the appearance of the rash.

22. DE

Duchenne muscular dystrophy is an x-linked autosomal recessive condition. Females are asymptomatic carriers. Learning disability is seen in about 20% of cases. There is an early delay in the motor milestones, and progressive muscular weakness. About 90% of boys are wheelchair dependent by 12 years. There may be cardiomyopathy and respiratory failure. Diagnosis is with a high plasma creatinine kinase and absent dystrophin on muscle biopsy.

23. ABE

Infantile spasms usually present within the first 12 months of life. There is equal incidence in males and females. The electroencephalogram shows disorganised hypsarrhythmia. It presents with Salam attacks which involve brief sudden flexion of the head, trunk and arms, lasting for a few seconds but can occur several times. It can be idiopathic, or associated with perinatal hypoxia, inborn errors of metabolism and tuberous sclerosis. It may lead to developmental regression.

24. AE

Absence seizures show bursts of 3cycles per second spike and wave activity on the electroencephalogram (EEG). Infantile spasms are associated with a disorganised hypsarrhythmia on electroencephalogram. Complex partial seizures are characterised by stereotypical behaviour and loss of consciousness. Benign rolandic epilepsy is characterised by nocturnal partial seizures and is linked to sudden unexplained death in epilepsy.

25. ACDE

At 12 months a normally developing child can say two words with meaning. Echolalia is normal at 15 months. At 18 months, they can follow a one-step command and point to parts of the body. At 2 years, they follow a two-step request and can identify objects from hearing their name. At three years they can say 3 to 4 word sentences, and are singing nursery rhymes. At 4 years they can count to 10 and can identify several colours.

26. BE

According to the British Thoracic Society Guidelines for asthma management; Step 1 involves the use of a short acting bronchodilator as needed. Step 2 is the addition of a low dose inhaled steroid, or other preventive drug if a steroid inhaler cannot be taken. Step three: in children under five years, a leukotriene antagonist is added; in over five year olds, a long acting bronchodilator and increased dose steroid inhaler are used, and if still not controlled then slow release theophylline or a leukotriene antagonist can be added. At step 4, the steroid inhaler is increased. Step five involves the use of oral steroids and referral to a respiratory paediatrician. Treatment can be started at any step which is most appropriate to the condition the child is at. Drug compliance should be checked before stepping up treatment, and stepping down treatment when control is achieved should be discussed with the patient and parents. The Turbohaler is appropriate for use in children over five years.

27. BE

Squints occur in approximately 4% of children. There is a strong familial incidence. A non-paralytic squint is the most common form; it may be due to an underlying defect for example cataract, retinoblastoma, visual defects and retinopathy of prematurity. In the cover test, if the uncovered eye moves to fix on the object, it is a manifest squint. Without treatment a squint can lead to amblyopia. A latent squint is usually seen during illness or when the child is tired or stressed.

28. BCE

Depression and deliberate self-harm, are more common in females; whereas suicide is more common in males. Depression may present with psychosomatic symptoms like headache and abdominal pain, and there may be secondary enuresis. According to the Office of National Statistics; suicide is the third leading cause of death in adolescence after accidents and homicide.

29. ABCD

The BCG vaccine is a live vaccine and is contraindicated in children on oral steroids, treatment for malignant disease with chemotherapy and radiotherapy or bone marrow transplant within the last six months, and immunoglobulin treatment within the last three months, and those with Di George syndrome. Vaccination may result in disseminated disease in immunocompromised children.

30. ABC

Club foot or congenital talipes, is a developmental deformity of the foot, in which the foot points downwards and inwards. It occurs in one in 1000 live births. It is common in males with a male to female ratio of 2:1. It can be genetically inherited, although there are no known causes. It can be positional talipes; where the deformity is passive and rigid, but can be corrected. But in club foot, the deformity cannot be passively corrected. About 50% are bilateral. A full neurological examination is required, as it may be associated with cerebral palsy or spina bifida. Serial splinting or casting helps, but some cases may need surgical treatment.

31. ABC

Signs of physical abuse include bruises of different ages, especially on the head, face, back, wrists, ankles and around the ears. A perforated eardrum can result from being hit on the side of the head. Spiral fractures of the humerus can be due to physical abuse, as can femoral fractures, in children who are not yet walking independently. A torn frenulum may be seen as a result of a blow to the mouth or force feeding with a bottle.

32. AE

Only 5% of children with faltering growth have an organic cause. A fall through two centiles or weight or height less than the second centile needs to be investigated. Recent research has shown that socio-economic disadvantage and neglect are not commonly associated with faltering growth. According to NICE, healthy babies should be weighed at birth, 8, 12 and 16 weeks and at one year. If there are any concerns, then once a month up to 6 months, then every two months from 6 to 12 months.

33. DE

Attention deficit hyperactivity disorder (ADHD) occurs in up to 3% of school age children. The diagnostic criteria include: inattention, hyperactivity and impulsiveness. It is more common in boys, with a male to female ratio of 5:1. Intelligence is usually normal but performance is reduced at school compared to peers, leading to significant impairment in social or academic development. Learning disability and disturbance in language and comprehension is associated with autism. Stereotypical behaviour is seen in Asperger's syndrome. ADHD is associated with food additives such as tartrazine, E102, sunset yellow, E110, Carmoisine, E122 and amaranth.

34. ABCDE

The following are notifiable diseases: measles, mumps, rubella, smallpox, yellow fever, polio, tetanus, whooping cough, cholera, diphtheria, acute infectious hepatitis, acute meningitis, acute encephalitis, typhoid, paratyphoid, food poisoning, legionnaire's disease, leprosy and malaria. HIV is not a notifiable disease.

35. ABCE

Obesity can be caused by a deficiency of growth hormone. It is associated with Down's syndrome, Prader-Willi syndrome and Lawrence-Moon-Biedl syndrome. It is associated with hyperinsulinism and diabetes.

36. ABCD

Coeliac serology should be considered in the investigation of constipation. Biopsy may be needed in diagnosing Hirschsprung's disease, in which there is absence of ganglion cells in the myenteric plexus in the rectum, and may be associated with Down's syndrome. Laxatives can be used long term, they are often needed in children who are toilet training, and should continue till bowel movements are well-established.

37. AD

Phenylketonuria has a carrier rate of one in 50 and incidence of one in 10,000 in the UK. Untreated it leads to developmental delay in the first year, learning disability and behavioural problems. There is decreased pigmentation, photosensitivity and dry skin. Dietary restriction is the mainstay of treatment. Phenylalanine is teratogenic and can harm the fetus, therefore strict dietary control is needed preconception and during pregnancy.

38. A

Primary teeth begin to appear between six months to one year of age. All natal teeth should be assessed by a dentist and be removed if loose or if they interfere with feeding. During teething the gums maybe sore and red where the tooth is coming out, and the baby may chew a lot or dribble and is irritable. Hutchinson's teeth, with notched incisors occur in congenital syphilis.

39. AC

Nitrofurantoin increases the risk of haemolytic anaemia in neonates and in glucose-6-phosphate dehydrogenase deficient infants. Sulphasalazine can precipitate kernicterus in babies.

40. ACD

Primary prevention programs are designed to reduce the incidence of new cases of disease presenting within the community. Some examples are immunisation, reducing parental smoking, preventing accidents and poisoning, breast-feeding promotion to improve nutrition, and the back to sleep program for prevention of cot death and sudden infant death, preventing dental disease and child abuse. Secondary prevention programs reduce the prevalence of disease, such as the blood spot test to detect hypothyroidism, phenylketonuria and cystic fibrosis, and the newborn hearing screen.

41. ABE

Noonan syndrome and Cushing syndrome are associated with short stature.

42. ABE

Atopic eczema usually presents in the first six months of life. 50% resolve by six years. It is associated with asthma, food intolerance and allergy. Antihistamines may be useful for sedation in acute exacerbations with sleep disturbance.

43. CDE

The evidence for use of bronchodilators in acute bronchiolitis is not strong, but Atrovent is used often with success. Acute bronchiolitis is caused by the respiratory syncytial virus in over 70% of cases. Other causes include Adenovirus, Para- influenza, rhinovirus, mumps, influenza and Mycoplasma pneumonia. It is most common under two years. No active vaccine is currently available.

44. D

Cot death or Sudden Infant Death Syndrome (SIDS) is the sudden, unexpected and unexplained death of a baby under one year. The highest incidence of cot death is between 2 and 4 months of age. Protective factors include: sleeping supine, sleeping as promoted in the back to sleep campaign, separate cot, appropriate room temperature, and a pacifier prevents deep sleeping; stopping smoking significantly reduces the incidence of cot death, whereas apnoea monitors do not.

45. ACE

Autism usually develops before three years of age. It may present with disturbance of communication including language comprehension and expression. IQ is reduced; normal intelligence may be seen in Asperger's and ADHD.

46. ABE

Gastro-oesophageal reflux is caused by delayed gastric emptying and is associated with liquid diets. It may present with dystonic posture as in Sandifer's syndrome.

47. ABDE

Precocious puberty is defined as signs of puberty less than eight years in girls, and under nine years in boys. In girls often no underlying cause is found, whereas it is almost always pathological in boys. Premature thelarche is usually seen in girls between 1 to 3 years. Precocious puberty initially leads to tall stature, but the child eventually ends up short, due to the premature closure of the epiphyses. Gonadotropin hormone releasing hormone analogues are used to stop the progression of puberty, by achieving non-pulsatile levels which lead to the suppression of the secretion of gonadotropins from the pituitary.

48. ACE

The vertical transmission rate of HIV with no intervention is 15 to 30%; however according to the WHO, this can be reduced to 2 % with efficacious interventions. All children under two years should be started on triple antiretroviral treatment. Children between 2 to 5 years with a CD4 count less than 25%, or an absolute count of less than 750 cells/mm3 require antiretroviral treatment, whereas children over five years with an absolute CD4 count of less than 350 cells/mm3 require treatment. Both HIV and AIDS are not notifiable to the Department of Public Health, but all children with HIV infection, and all infants born to HIV positive mothers in the UK should be reported to the British Paediatric Surveillance Unit (BPSU) at the UCL (University College London)-Institute of Child Health. Vaginal delivery is allowed for patients who are well-controlled on treatment, and with good CD4 counts and undetectable viral loads.

49. ABCDE

Rickets occurs due to decreased serum calcium, which leads to growth abnormalities, short stature, frontal bossing, delayed dentition, enlarged costal cartilages, deformities of the lower limbs, widened epiphyseal regions in long bones and delayed weight-bearing milestones.

50. BCE

Non-accidental head injury is most commonly seen in infants less than six months. It can result in the development of intracranial haemorrhage which is typically subdural, subarachnoid and intra ventricular haemorrhage. Extradural haemorrhage is rare. There may be brain injury, skull fractures, retinal haemorrhage and bruising. Bilateral black eyes may indicate blood tracking down after significant injury to the forehead.

51. CE

The MMR vaccine should not be given to children who have had a bone marrow transplant, chemotherapy or radiotherapy within six months, or immunoglobulins within three months. It can be given to most children who have had allergic reactions to eggs, and should be given in controlled conditions to those with confirmed anaphylaxis. It may lead to parotid swelling in up to 1% of cases. It is contraindicated in children allergic to neomycin and kanamycin. ITP (Idiopathic Thrombocytopenic Purpura) may occur in 1 in 22,000 children within six weeks of the first dose of the MMR. It resolves spontaneously. Arthropathy occurs rarely 2 to 3 weeks after the immunisation.

52. BD

Cystic fibrosis has a carrier frequency of 1:25, leading to disease in 1:2500 births of white babies. The lungs are normal at birth. Up to 30 percent of cases have nasal polyps. Cystic fibrosis is associated with meconium ileus, rectal prolapse, malabsorption, delayed puberty and diabetes mellitus.

53. ABC

Tinea corporis causes annular lesions with central clearing on the face, limbs and trunk. Tinea capitis causes patchy dandruff-like scaling with hair loss and discrete pustules or kerion formation. It shows up as fluorescent green on Wood's light. Topical agents are not effective, and treatment with oral antifungals such as

Griseofulvin or Terbinafine is required. Tinea pedis usually responds to topical antifungal agents.

54. CE

Incidence is the total number of new cases in a population, whereas prevalence is the total number of cases in the population at any one time. Specificity is the percentage of those who do not have a condition who are correctly tested negative, whereas sensitivity is the percentage of those who have the condition and are correctly tested positive. A statistically significant result may not be clinically significant, and therefore other factors should be considered, such as in the case of drugs consider costs, side-effects, improvement in the problem, administration etc.

55. ABE

Coxsackie virus A16 causes hand foot and mouth disease. Glandular fever is caused by Epstein-Barr virus, there is no cure, and the treatment is symptomatic. It can be confused with a bacterial throat infection, and if treated with amoxicillin can lead to a maculopapular rash, which can be mistaken for an allergic reaction. The Epstein – Barr virus affects B lymphocytes.

56. CDE

Non-gastrointestinal manifestations of coeliac disease include alopecia, anaemia, fatigue, faltering growth, delayed puberty and short stature. Migraine, rickets, stomatitis and dermatitis herpetiformis may be present as well as amenorrhoea and neuropathies.

57. ABD

Neonatal acne is due to maternal androgens and usually resolves by three months. Investigation is needed if the initial presentation is before puberty, to exclude endocrine abnormalities such as, Cushing's syndrome, diabetes, virilising tumours and polycystic ovaries. Boys are more commonly affected than girls. Acne is caused by the anaerobic Propionibacterium acnes, which causes infection within the follicle. Isotretinoin (Roaccutane) is a vitamin A derivative, which is started by a specialist only. It needs monitoring with lipid and liver function tests. It is teratogenic and therefore contraception is needed, it can cause depression.

58. CDE

Parental consent is needed for a child up to 16 years; between 16 to 18 years it is needed if the young person is incapacitated. Under English law, a child cannot refuse treatment for serious conditions. Preschool children are unable to provide valid consent, but they should be involved in the process, and their questions must be answered. A 14-year-old has the right to confidentiality, under Fraser guidelines eg. contraception. An unmarried father cannot consent to treatment for his child, unless if he has formal agreement with the mother or court.

59. AB

Referred pain from the abdomen, for example, due to appendicitis, inguinal hernia and urinary tract infection, may cause hip pain. Septic arthritis commonly affects the hip and knee joints. The peak age at presentation is three years, but can affect children of any age. Irritable hip commonly affects children aged 1 to 4 years. Perthes disease is due to avascular necrosis of the femoral head. It is bilateral in 15%. Irritable hip is an idiopathic benign inflammation, and is a common cause of admission to hospital. Investigations are normal, it usually resolves spontaneously.

60. ACDE

According to the WHO (2009), breastfeeding reduces the incidence of respiratory and gastrointestinal tract infections, and atopic eczema. Babies who are breastfed have a reduced risk of developing diabetes, childhood leukaemia and lymphomas and obesity in adolescence. Breastfeeding reduces the incidence of ear and throat infections.

Answers Paper 5

The following statements are true.

1. BDE

The characteristic sub- occipital lymphadenopathy in Rubella appears 24 hours before the rash. Retro-auricular and posterior cervical lymph nodes may be involved. Infection in the first eight weeks of gestation results in severe abnormality or fetal death. Hydrocephalus and calcification in the brain are characteristically seen in cytomegalovirus and toxoplasmosis infection. Sensorineural hearing loss and microcephaly are seen in Rubella. Typically congenital rubella causes microphthalmia, micro cornea, anterior uveitis, cataract and glaucoma. The rash begins on the trunk and spreads to the face.

2. ABE

There is normal learning ability in Turner's syndrome and achondroplasia.

3. D

Homocystinuria is associated with developmental delay and reduced intelligence. There is normal to tall marfanoid habitus, stiff joints and osteoporosis. Downward subluxation of the lens is seen in Homocystinuria, whereas upward subluxation is seen in Marfan's syndrome.

4. BCD

Breath-holding attacks are seen in young children under the age of five. The child cries and holds their breath becoming cyanosed and may have a convulsion. Reflex anoxic seizures are precipitated by a sudden unexpected painful stimulus or by vomiting. This leads to the stimulation of the Vagus nerve, causing bradycardia, pallor, collapse and convulsions, followed by spontaneous recovery. They usually improve with age, but may persist. Psychogenic seizures are under conscious or subconscious control. They are usually triggered by psychological disturbance. There may be sudden collapse and convulsions. The child may respond to their surroundings. Management is by psychological counselling. Myoclonic seizures lead to sudden muscular jerks.

5. ABDE

Maternal diabetes leads to fetal macrosomia, neonatal hypoglycaemia, hypomagnesaemia, hypocalcaemia and polycythaemia. Other associations are cardiac defects including aortic coarctation, transposition of the great arteries and septal defects, sacral agenesis, short femur, renal agenesis and imperforate anus.

6. ABCE

The differential diagnosis of non-accidental fractures includes: accidental injury, osteopenia, vitamin deficiencies, malignancy and infection.

7. ABCD

Parental factors predisposing to abuse include; young parents with poor relationship, drug abuse, history of abuse in their childhood, domestic violence, deprivation, lower social class, mental illness, learning disability and difficult pregnancy. Predisposing factors from the child include: pre-maturity, admission to the special care baby unit, difficult behaviour and physical and learning disabilities.

8. DE

Egg-on- side cardiac outline is seen in transposition of the great arteries. Oligaemic lung fields are due to reduced pulmonary blood flow, and are seen in tetralogy of Fallot, Ebstein's anomaly and pulmonary hypertension. Boot- shaped heart is seen in tetralogy of Fallot.

9. BCE

The Q-T interval on ECG is prolonged if it is more than 0.44 seconds in a child more than six months. It varies with the heart rate. In infants less than six months up to 0.49 seconds is normal. It may be congenital, and is seen in hypokalaemia, hypocalcaemia, hypomagnesaemia and hypothermia, head injury with raised intra-cranial pressure, in the long QT syndrome, Romano –Ward syndrome and drugs.

10. All false

A normal PR interval in children is 0.08-0.16 seconds. Atrial septal defects, myocarditis, digoxin toxicity and hyperkalaemia, are causes of a long P-R interval. Erythromycin causes a long Q-T interval.

11. ABD

The incidence of rheumatic fever in the UK is increasing, due to the reduced use of antibiotics for sore throats. A history of streptococcal throat infection and two major criteria, or one major, and two minor are required for diagnosis. The presence of subcutaneous nodules is one of the major diagnostic criteria for rheumatic fever. Others include: erythema marginatum, carditis, polyarthritis and chorea. The minor criteria are: raised white cells, CRP or ESR, arthralgia, past history of rheumatic fever or rheumatic heart disease and prolonged PR interval on ECG.

12. ABD

80-90% of small ventricular septal defects are asymptomatic. Large defects maybe symptomatic with heart failure after one week of life. Tetralogy of Fallot should be repaired at 6 to 9 months of age. Atrial septal defects (ASD) should be closed at 3 to 5 years. ECG findings in ASD include: prolonged PR interval, in ostium primum defects there is a left axis deviation of the QRS complex, and in ostium secundum there is a right axis deviation.

13. ABDE

Maternal diabetes can lead to polycythaemia in the infant.

14. ABCE

Toe-walking is common between the ages of 1 to 2 years, but if it persists beyond 3 years, a neurological examination is required. It may be idiopathic. Other causes include pre-maturity, spastic cerebral palsy, congenital shortening of the Achilles tendon, spinal tumour and unilateral hip dislocation. Spina bifida is associated with talipes.

15. D

The overlying skin is normal in cephalhaematoma and is bruised and oedematous in caput succedaneum. Cephalhaematoma usually resolves over a few weeks, whereas caput disappears over a few days.

Cephalhaematoma appears a few hours after birth, and may require phototherapy for jaundice if large.

16. BD

The aetiology of Kawasaki disease is unknown. There is a systemic vasculitis with fever for more than five days, rash, conjunctivitis and cervical lymphadenopathy. Thrombocytosis occurs later in the sub-acute phase at the end of the second week. Management is with aspirin and intravenous immunoglobulins. Mortality is 1-2% and is usually due to cardiac complications, like myocarditis or infarction.

17. ABCE

Cafe -a- lait spots can be idiopathic, familial, congenital naevus, and are associated with ataxia telangiectasia, neurofibromatosis, McCune Albright syndrome, Bloom syndrome and Gaucher's disease.

18. ABDE

Macrocephaly maybe caused by meningitis which may also cause microcephaly. Other causes include hydrocephalus, chronic subdural haematoma, meningeal malignancy, genetic, Soto's syndrome, achondroplasia, tuberous sclerosis, mucopolysaccharidosis, incontinentia pigmenti, rickets, renal disease and osteogenesis imperfecta. There is microcephaly in Trisomy 13 or Patau's syndrome.

19. ABCDE

Hypotonia is seen in the early stages of kernicterus, and in birth asphyxia leading to hypotonic cerebral palsy. Trisomy 13, 18 and 21 can present with hypotonia.

20. ABE

In insulin-dependent diabetes there may be delayed puberty, short stature and retinopathy. It is associated with coeliac disease, autoimmune thyroid disease and Addison's disease.

21. ABCDE

Xeroderma pigmentosa is associated with increased risk of skin cancer. Klinefelter's syndrome is associated with breast cancer. There is increased risk of central nervous system tumours in 5 to 10% of cases of neurofibromatosis. In coeliac disease, if a gluten-free diet is not adhered to, there is an increased risk of gastrointestinal malignancy. Down's syndrome is associated with increased risk of leukaemia.

22. ABCE

Undescended testes are common in preterm babies. At 30 weeks, it is seen in 20-50 % and in 2-5 % at term. It is associated with myotonic dystrophy and Kallmann's syndrome. Klinefelter's syndrome is associated with small testes.

23. AE

Gilbert syndrome is autosomal recessive but can be autosomal dominant with incomplete expression. It is more common in males, and may lead to breast milk and neonatal jaundice. There is unconjugated hyperbilirubinaemia.

24. ABCDE

Down's syndrome is associated with cardiac defects such as ventriculoseptal defect, atrioventricular septal defect and patents ductus arteriosus. There may be gastrointestinal defects such as, oesophageal atresia, duodenal atresia, Hirschsprung's disease and coeliac disease. Other associations are cataract, leukaemia and Alzheimer's disease.

25. BC

School refusal is seen equally in boys and girls. It is seen in high achievers, and is due to an anxiety regarding school attendance, in contrast to truancy which may be a part of a conduct disorder, and reflects a lack of desire to go to school.

26. A

Sleeping with parents may be a contributing factor to sleep difficulties in children. Behavioural strategies are usually more successful than sedating antihistamines. Nightmares occur in 25 to 50% of children aged 3 to 5 years, and maybe associated with anxiety. Sleepwalking occurs in stages three or four of sleep and is most often seen in 8 to 14 year olds.

27. BE

Strawberry naevi appear in the first few weeks of life, and may grow over the next 6 to 10 months before undergoing spontaneous resolution; whereas port wine stains are present at birth and usually persist throughout life, they are associated with the Sturge-Weber syndrome.

28. D

Lactose intolerance is usually acquired most commonly after a rotavirus infection. Radioallergosorbent testing (RAST) lacks sensitivity or specificity for diagnosing cow's milk allergy. Children with early-onset allergy to peanuts may grow out of it; and allergy in older children is more likely to continue. Soya products should not be used in infants less than six months of age, due to the presence of phyto- oestrogens in soya milk. There is cross-reactivity between cow's milk and soya protein; therefore hydrolysed formula should be used in children intolerant to cow's milk.

29. AE

Unilateral wheeze is seen on clinical examination in foreign body inhalation, due to reduced air entry. Peanuts are radiolucent and do not show up on chest x-ray. Removal of the foreign body under bronchoscopy is needed, especially in peanuts, as they may cause inflammation and airway narrowing leading to lobar collapse.

30. BDE

Umbilical herniae usually close spontaneously by five years of age, whereas supra-umbilical herniae require surgical closure.

31. ABCE

Antenatal diagnosis by amniocenteses is used to diagnose autosomal recessive and sex-linked recessive conditions, neural tube defects and genetic syndromes. Gastroschisis is diagnosed on ultrasound scan.

32. ABC

There is increased risk of neurodevelopmental problems as a complication of intrauterine growth retardation.

33. ACE

Inspiratory stridor due to laryngomalacia worsens in the supine position, with crying, and upper respiratory tract infections. It can lead to faltering growth due to recurrent apnoea in which case, referral for an upper airway endoscopy is required, otherwise it usually resolves by two years.

34. ADE

Cystic hygroma is a congenital lesion, but may not be obvious at birth. It is noticed when it increases in size in upper respiratory tract infection, after which it usually involutes. It is commonly found in the neck, and is brilliantly transilluminating on examination. It is diagnosed by ultrasound scan, and a CT scan maybe needed to define the extent. Surgical excision may be required for large lesions. It is associated with Turner syndrome and Noonan syndrome.

35. BC

Hypospadias occurs in one in 300 live births. The aetiology is unknown; however it is associated with deficiency of testosterone secretion or responsiveness, and disorders of sexual differentiation. Circumcision should not be performed, as tissue may be required for corrective surgery. Severe forms, for example peno-scrotal and perineal hypospadias are associated with renal tract anomalies.

36. BC

Methylphenidate is used for children over the age of six years, with severe ADHD as part of a comprehensive treatment plan. Treatment should be started and monitored by child psychiatrists or paediatricians with expertise in ADHD, GPs can share care. Side- effects include: weight and growth retardation and hypertension; therefore, six -monthly monitoring of height, weight, pulse and blood pressure is needed. Drug treatment does not cure ADHD, but improves the symptoms allowing other interventions to work.

37. ABE

Poor prognostic signs in acute lymphoblastic leukaemia include: age less than two years or over nine years, male sex, African Caribbean ethnicity, and central nervous system disease, because lymphoblasts can be protected from chemotherapy by the blood brain barrier.

38. ABE

Micturating cystourethrogram is used to diagnose vesico-ureteric reflux, which can aid in grading according to severity. Reflux nephropathy leads to renal failure in 15 to 20% of cases. Long-term antibiotic prophylaxis is needed, however in uncomplicated cases there is little benefit in continuing over five years.

39. ABD

Hyperthyroidism and coarctation of the aorta can cause hypertension, as well as reflux nephropathy, chronic renal failure, polycystic kidney disease, glomerulonephritis, renal artery stenosis, Wilm's tumour, raised intracranial pressure, phaeochromocytoma, Cushing's syndrome and steroids.

40. All false

The onset of myasthenia gravis is usually after one year. Adolescent girls are more commonly affected. The extra- ocular muscles are affected earlier in the disease and proximal limb and bulbar muscles are involved later.

41. BE

Neck stiffness rarely occurs in meningitis in neonates. It usually presents with non-specific signs and symptoms. Neurological sequelae maybe seen in up to 30% of children; and include, neurological deficits, learning disability, hydrocephalus and deafness. The head circumference must be monitored as there may be subdural effusions and hydrocephalus.

42. ABDE

Vitamin D deficiency is seen in exclusive breastfeeding of 6 to 12 months. Vitamin D deficiency leads to decreased calcium absorption, low plasma calcium, high alkaline phosphatase and increased parathyroid hormone levels. Vitamin D requires hydroxylation in the liver and kidney to its active form, therefore liver and renal disease can lead to low levels of vitamin D. Deficiency is very common in the UK, and primary prevention with vitamins for high risk groups, including children and pregnant women is justified.

43. ABD

A white pupillary reflex or absent red reflex requires referral. It is also seen in uveitis, vitreous haemorrhage, and coloboma and Toxocara infections.

44. ABC

Schizophrenia is rare in childhood. It is more common in boys, and is associated with perinatal illness and psychosocial factors. It can be confused with physical disease; therefore any child with a psychotic episode should have an electro encephalogram and MRI scan of the brain. Acute onset is associated with a better prognosis, as is older age at onset and high intelligence.

45. ABCDE

Organic causes of psychosis include, neurodegenerative diseases, thyrotoxicosis and drug induced psychosis.

46. AD

The mean age of presentation of dermatitis herpetiformis is 7 years. It typically affects the buttocks, elbows, neck and scalp. Bullous pemphigoid can be seen in children less than 12 months. 75% have mucous membrane involvement. It lasts for 2 to 4 years. Nikolsky's sign is positive in pemphigus, and is seen on rubbing normal skin, which leads to blister formation.

47. ABCDE

Non-gastrointestinal manifestations of coeliac disease include: rickets, osteoporosis and osteomalacia, iron deficiency anaemia, fatigue, delayed puberty, short stature, faltering growth, irritability, neuropathies, and ataxia and dermatitis herpetiformis.

48. E

Developmental dysplasia of the hip (DDH) occurs in 2 in 1000. It is more common in females, with a female to male ratio of 5:1. Other risk factors include; family history, breech presentation, and is common in first born children. Ortolani's test is abducting the dislocated hip to reduce it. Barlow's test involves adducting and depressing the femur. Both tests are unreliable after 6 to 8 weeks. The older child presents with a painless limp, and a positive Trendelenberg test.

49. AE

Nocturnal enuresis can be a sign of sexual abuse. Lifting and waking, and dry bed training with or without an alarm have not been shown to help. Desmopressin can be used in children over seven years.

50. BD

Meningococcal serogroup B is the most common important infectious cause of death in children in the UK, and there is no vaccine for it. The highest incidence is in children under two years, with another peak in adolescence and early adulthood. The fatality rate of meningitis is 10%. Benzyl penicillin should be used in patients suspected to have meningococcal meningitis or if urgent transfer to hospital is not possible due to remote location, or adverse weather. The dose of Benzyl penicillin in adults and children over 10 years is 1200 mg IV or IM. In children 1 to 9 years is 600 mg in infants 300 mg. Ciprofloxacin is recommended for chemoprophylaxis in all ages. It is given as a single dose.

51. BE

Encopresis is defined as inappropriate passage of faeces into the underwear after the age of four years. Physical problems such as hypothyroidism, Hirschsprung disease and hypercalcaemia may lead to encopresis. It usually resolves during childhood.

52. BCE

The neonatal blood spot test is done on day 6. The Guthrie test may be false-negative if the child is on antibiotics, as it relies on phenylalanine- dependent bacterial growth. The neonatal blood spot test screens for hypothyroidism, phenylketonuria, sickle cell disease, MCADD (Medium Chain Acyl Dehydrogenase Deficiency), Maple Syrup urine disease (MSUD), isovaleric acidaemia (IVA), glutaric aciduria type 1 (GA1), homocystinuria and cystic fibrosis.

53. BDE

Obesity in children can result from growth hormone deficiency due to hypopituitarism, hypogonadism and hypothyroidism. It is associated with Down's syndrome, and can be monogenic and iatrogenic due to steroids.

54. BDE

The mother automatically has parental responsibility, however the father has parental responsibility if he was married to the mother at the time of the child's birth, or if they were unmarried but his name was registered on the birth certificate after December 2003. An unmarried father may gain parental responsibility, if he enters into a parental responsibility agreement with the mother, or if he has a court order. The biological parents lose parental responsibility on adoption of the child, or if the child is awarded to the local authority as part of an emergency protection order or care order.

55. ABCD

NICE advises to consider screening for coeliac disease in patients with; depression, bipolar disorder, Down's syndrome (5-12% incidence), Turner syndrome (6-8% incidence), lymphoma, osteomalacia, sarcoidosis, Addison's disease, polyneuropathy and in persistently raised unexplained liver enzymes.

56. BCE

Eating disorders are more prevalent in higher social classes. Patients may have dry skin and lanugo hair, muscle aches, osteoporosis and pathological fractures. The mortality rate is between 5 to 20%. Cause of death is usually from starvation, electrolyte imbalance, heart failure and suicide.

57. BDE

There is increased incidence of surfactant deficiency in prematurity, males, maternal diabetes, elective Caesarean section, sepsis, second twin, and a positive family history. It is reduced in females, maternal opiate use and antenatal steroids.

58. CD

Retinoblastoma may be sporadic or familial. There is a positive family history in up to 25% of cases. The most common age of diagnosis is between 12 to 18 months, 80% are diagnosed before the age of three years. It usually presents with leukocoria or absent light reflex in 60%, visual deterioration, and squint. Treatment is with surgery, chemotherapy and radiotherapy. The five-year survival rate is 90%; however long-term follow up is needed, as the inherited form is at risk of a second primary malignancy, most commonly an osteosarcoma.

59. CD

The most common cause of viral meningitis is Enterovirus followed by Herpes simplex virus. Encephalitis peaks in the first 6 months of life and is predominantly viral in origin. In bacterial meningitis, the cerebrospinal fluid protein level is raised to more than 0.4g/l and glucose is reduced. The white-cell count is raised to more than 1000/mm3. In older children headache followed by neck stiffness occurs within 12 to 24 hours, but is often absent in infants, and a lumbar puncture should be considered for any infant with unexplained fever. The data supporting the use of steroids is weak, however some studies show that steroids may reduce the severity of neurological sequelae and deafness .Mycobacterium tuberculosis affects children of all ages.

60. B

Diurnal enuresis is much more common in girls. Enuresis is associated with psychiatric illness in 25% of children. According to NICE guidance CG111, alarms should be the first line of treatment in children who have not responded to advice on fluids, toileting or rewards. Urinalysis should not be done routinely, but should be considered if the child has recently started bedwetting, if there are daytime symptoms, any signs of ill health, history of, or signs and symptoms of a urinary tract infection or diabetes mellitus. Lifting and waking the child is not advised. Drug treatment with desmopressin should be considered in children over the age of seven years. Sexual abuse must be considered in any child presenting with enuresis or encopresis.

Bibliography

BNF for Children 2016/17

British Thoracic Society Guidelines 2016 www.brit-thoracic.org.uk

www.dermnetnz.org

NICE Guidance

Office for National Statistics www.ons.gov.uk

World Health Organisation www.who.int

http://www.nhs.uk/

RCPCH Guidelines

Oxford Handbook of Paediatrics 2013

Nelson's Textbook of Paediatrics, 20 th Edition

Illustrated Textbook of Paediatrics, 4th Edition Lissauer, Clayden

Essential Revision Notes in Paediatrics for the MRCPCH, 3 rd Edition, Beattie, Champion

www.gpnotebook.co.uk

Health Protection Agency-Gov.uk

The Green Book: Immunisation against Infectious diseases 2014

Public Health England-Gov.uk

NHS Screening www.cpd.screening.nhs.uk

Children Act 1989 www.legislation.gov.uk>1989

Parental Rights and Responsibilities-Gov.uk

Department of Health –Gov.uk

NCPCC www.nspc.org.uk

Ofsted www.gov.uk

Index

A

Abdominal migraine 79, 207

Abdominal pain 78, 79, 141, 144, 206, 207

Absence seizures 24, 25, 85, 148, 149, 212

Accidental poisoning 41

Achondroplasia 26, 100, 102, 150, 192, 227, 232

Acne 98, 225

Acrodermatitis enteropathica 41, 166

Activated charcoal 42, 167

Acute lymphoblastic leukaemia 51, 113, 177, 178, 238

Adenoma sebaceum 18, 139, 188

ADHD 113, 127, 216, 220, 238

Alagilles's syndrome 44, 170

Alpha-1 antitrypsin deficiency 43, 170, 199, 208, 211

Alternating squints 16, 137

Amblyopia 16, 136, 137, 214

Amniocentesis 111, 236

Angelman syndrome 27, 152

Anorexia nervosa 6, 30, 125

Antiepileptic drugs 26, 150

Aortic stenosis 76, 153, 203

Asthma 78, 86, 206, 213,

Ataxic cerebral palsy 57, 183

Ataxia telangiectasia 57, 184, 232

Atopic eczema 92, 219

Atrial septal defect 6, 11, 75, 104, 125, 153, 202, 231

Attention deficit hyperactivity disorder 89, 216

Autism 89, 93, 216, 220, 89

Autoimmune hepatitis 44, 171

Autosomal recessive inheritance 72, 199, 236

B

Back to sleep program 92, 219

Balanitis xerotica obliterans 20, 142

Barlow's test 118, 242

BCG 88, 215

Beckwith- Wiedemann syndrome 50, 56, 177, 179

Behavioural problems 17, 139, 193, 218

Bell's palsy 61, 187

Benign rolandic epilepsy 25, 86, 149, 213

Birthmarks 109, 235

Bone tumours 54, 180

Boot-shaped heart 30, 103

Breastfeeding 59, 185, 226, 240

Bronchiectasis 7, 126

Bronchiolitis 93, 219

Bullous pemphigoid 117, 241

Buphthalmos 18

C

Café au lait patches 62

Candida 41, 166

Capillary haemangioma 39, 164, 165

Carbamazepine 26, 150

Cardiac surgical mortality 29, 154

Case-control studies 13, 134

Cavernous haemangioma 39

Cephalhaematoma 105, 231

Cerebral haemorrhage 58, 173

Cerebral palsy 11, 23, 24, 56, 57, 146, 147, 173, 182

Cevarix 73, 200

Chicken pox 84, 211

Child abuse 8, 127

Child Assessment Order 9, 129

Childhood tics 66, 192

Child protection process 9, 129

Child protection review 10, 130

Children's Act 9

Chronic lung disease of prematurity 47, 126, 174

Cirrhosis 44, 171

Claw hand 62

Cleft lip/ palate 49, 175

Clubfoot 88, 198

Coarctation of the aorta 6, 104, 125, 160

Coeliac disease 43, 79, 98, 117, 121, 169, 207, 225, 241, 244

Cohort studies 13, 134

Complex partial seizures 86, 212

Conception rate 74, 201

Congenital adrenal hyperplasia 69, 196

Congenital heart disease 6, 29, 32, 104, 157

Congenital rubella 100, 227

Conjugated hyperbilirubinaemia 42

Consent 98, 225

Constipation 90, 217

Constitutional obesity 181, 195, 221

Co-operative language test 17

Cornelia de Lange syndrome 26

Cot death 93, 219, 220

Cover test 16

Coxsackie virus 97, 191, 224

Cross-sectional studies 13

Cryptorchidism 19, 28

Cystic fibrosis 7, 10, 78, 96, 126, 130, 206, 223

Cystic hygroma 112, 237

Cytomegalovirus 72, 199, 227

D

Delayed puberty 24, 147

Dentition 91, 218

Depression 87, 214

Dermatomyositis 62, 189

Developmental dysplasia of the hip 117, 198, 242

Developmental milestones 72, 199

Developmental regression 62, 85

Diabetes mellitus 59, 66, 101, 104, 107, 126, 141, 157, 184, 185, 193, 194, 206, 217, 223, 228, 231, 233, 247

Diaphragmatic hernia 48, 174

Di George's syndrome 32, 157

Diplegia 11, 23, 132, 147

Distraction test 17, 138

DNA viruses 74, 202

Down's syndrome 41, 108, 167, 234

Duchenne muscular dystrophy 73, 85, 199, 212

Dyskinetic cerebral palsy 57, 182

E

Early neonatal mortality rate 12, 133

Eating disorders 121, 245

EEG 25, 85, 121, 155, 212

Eisenmenger's syndrome 34, 159

Emergency protection order 9, 128

Encephalitis, 64, 65, 135, 246

Encopresis 119, 243

Enuresis 118, 122, 242, 246

Epidemiology 12

Epidermolysis bullosa 36, 162

Epilepsy 24, 25, 85, 147, 148, 149, 150, 212

Erythema multiforme 37, 163

Erythrasma 37, 163

Ewing's sarcoma 27, 54, 151, 180

Exchange transfusion 67, 194

Exomphalos 49, 176

Extradural haemorrhage 59, 185, 222

F

Faltering growth 89, 216

Fears and phobias 6, 126

Febrile convulsions 25, 149

Food allergies 110, 235

Foreign body inhalation 110, 236

Fragile X syndrome 27, 152

Friedreich's ataxia 33, 58, 183

G

Galactosaemia 67, 73, 106, 193, 199

Gardasil 73, 200

Gastric lavage 41, 167

Gastroesophageal reflux 94, 221

Gastroschisis 49, 176

Gilbert's syndrome 108, 234

Gingival fibromas 62, 188

Grasping reflex 84

Guillain- Barre Syndrome 60, 186

Guthrie test 81, 119, 127, 243, 217

Guttate psoriasis 36, 161

H

Haemangiomas 39, 164

Haemophilus influenza B vaccine 14, 135

Hair loss 40, 166

Hand preference 11, 132

Hearing loss 16, 137

Hearing screening 17, 138

Hemiplegia 11, 132, 147

Hepatitis B 44, 171

Hepatitis B immunisation 15, 136, 185

Hepatitis C 44, 171

Hepatitis D 44, 171

Henoch-Schonlein purpura 55, 181

Hereditary angioedema 38, 164

Herpes simplex virus 64, 190

Herpes virus 64, 162, 190

Heterophil antibodies 63, 190

Hip pain 69, 99, 196, 197, 226

HIV 94, 221

Hodgkin's disease 52, 178

Homocystinuria 100, 227, 243

Horner's syndrome 55, 182

HPV vaccine 73, 200

Hutchinson's teeth 91, 218

Hydrocephalus 22, 145

Hydrocoele 19, 141

Hypergammaglobulinaemia 171

Hypertension 35, 114, 160, 239

Hypogammaglobulinaemia 126, 184

Hypogonadotrophic hypogonadism 28, 153, 210

Hypospadias 113, 237

Hypotonia 106, 233

I

Idiopathic scrotal oedema 21, 142

Inborn errors of metabolism 66, 193,

Incidence 12, 13, 97, 132, 134, 219, 224

Infant mortality rate 12, 133

Infantile seborrhoeic dermatitis 38, 164

Infantile spasms 18, 25, 85, 139, 148, 212

Infectious mononucleosis 63, 190

Inguinal hernia 19, 140

Initial child protection case conference 9, 128

Innocent murmur 31, 156

Interferon 44

Intrauterine growth retardation 112, 170, 194, 237

Intussusception 21, 78, 144, 206

Irritable hip 69, 99, 196, 226

Irritant dermatitis 41, 166

J

Jaundice 42, 83, 108, 168, 169, 170, 194, 210, 234

Juvenile myasthenia 61, 187

Juvenile myoclonic epilepsy 25, 149

K

Kallmann's syndrome 28, 82, 153, 210, 234

Kawasaki disease 80, 105, 232

Kernicterus 47, 168, 174, 233

Koebner phenomenon 37, 162

L

Lactose intolerance 110, 235

Laryngomalacia 112, 237

Latent squint 16, 87, 137, 214

Lead poisoning 42, 167, 168

Learning disability 100

Leukocoria 54, 180, 245

Limit ages 77, 205

Lisch nodules 18, 140

Long PR interval 11, 58, 103, 131, 158, 184

Lumbar puncture 185, 246

Lyme disease 80, 208

Lymphoma 51, 177, 178

M

Macrocephaly, 65, 106, 192, 232

Malrotation 79, 206

Manifest squint 16, 137, 214

Marfan's syndrome 34, 160

Measles 14, 135

Meckel's diverticulum 79, 144, 206

Membranous nephropathy 53

Meningitis, 64, 65, 90, 115, 118, 122, 175, 190, 192, 208, 217, 232, 239, 242, 246

Meningocoele 22

Mesenteric adenitis 79, 206

Methylphenidate 8, 113, 127, 238

Minimal change disease 53

MMR 15, 96, 135, 223

Moro reflex 83

Mortality rates 12, 13

Mucopolysaccharidosis 39, 40, 62, 165, 189

Mumps 14, 64, 97, 135, 191, 202, 217, 220

Myasthenia gravis 114, 187, 239

Myelomeningocoele 22, 145

Myotonic dystrophy 63, 189, 199, 234

N

Necrotising enteropathic colitis 46, 173

Neglect 8, 127

Neonatal ECG 32, 157

Neonatal mortality rates 12, 133

Neonatal screening program 119, 243

Neonatal sepsis 48, 175

Nephrotic syndrome 53, 179

Notifiable diseases 89, 217

Neuroblastoma 51, 52, 177, 178

Neurofibromatosis 18, 61, 139, 188

Nikolsky's sign 117, 241

Nitric oxide 33, 159

N-myc oncogene 52

Non – accidental head injury 95, 222

Non-Hodgkin's lymphoma 52, 178

Noonan syndrome 22, 29, 32, 145, 153

O

Obesity 67, 68, 90, 120, 182, 194, 217, 243

Oesophageal atresia 50, 176

Orchitis 20, 142

Ortolani test 118, 242

Osteogenesis imperfecta 69, 196

Otoacoustic emissions 17, 138

P

Paraphimosis 20, 142

Parental responsibility 120, 244

Patent ductus arteriosus 31, 32, 34, 46, 157, 172

Pendred's syndrome 17, 137

Periventricular haemorrhage 46, 173

Periventricular leukomalacia 46, 173

Perthes disease 99, 197, 226

Pierre-Robin sequence 23, 49, 146, 175

Pityriasis rosea 36, 41, 162, 166

Phenylketonuria 67, 90, 193, 218, 219

Philadelphia chromosome 51, 113

Phimosis 20

Phototherapy 42, 83, 168, 211

Physical abuse 8, 31, 88, 127, 128, 156, 215

Pneumococcal vaccination 82, 209

Police protection order 9, 128

Positive likelihood ratio 97

Positive predictive value 14, 134

PR interval 58, 183

Prader- Willi syndrome 19, 20, 141

Precocious puberty 24, 68, 94, 195

Prevalence 12, 14, 132, 134

Primary prevention 81, 92, 209, 219

Primitive reflexes 83, 211

Prolonged QT syndrome 9, 30, 128, 156

Proteus 55, 181

Prune belly syndrome 54, 180

Psoriasis 36, 161

Pseudomonas 55, 181

Psychosis 116, 241

Puberty 24, 68, 147, 195

Pulmonary flow murmur 31, 157

Pulmonary stenosis 29, 153, 157, 158, 159, 203

Pyloric stenosis 21, 82, 143, 209

Q

Quadriplegia 11, 24, 132, 147

R

Red reflex 84, 211, 240

Reed Sternberg cells 52

Renal artery stenosis 35, 62, 188

Retinoblastoma 51, 54, 84, 116, 122, 180, 211, 245

Retinopathy of prematurity 47, 174

Rhabdomyomata 62, 188

Rheumatic fever 103, 230

Rickets 95, 222

Rifampicin 66, 192

Ring worm 96, 223

Rooting reflex 84, 211

Roseola infantum 64, 97, 190

Rubella 14, 15, 32, 100, 135, 157, 199, 202, 217, 227

S

Schizophrenia 116, 240

School phobia 7, 125

School refusal 109, 234

School sweep test 17

Screening for coeliac disease 60, 121, 244

Screening tests 13, 138

Secondary prevention 81, 219

Sensitivity 14, 97, 134, 224

Sensorineural hearing loss 16, 137

Separation anxiety 7, 125

Sexual abuse 8, 127, 242

Short stature 146, 233

Sickle cell disease 67, 81, 194, 209, 243

Skeletal survey 8, 127

Sleep apnoea 77, 130, 194, 205

Sleep problems 109, 235

Slipped upper femoral epiphysis 70, 71, 197

Smoking 92, 93, 201, 211, 219, 220

Snoring 10, 129

Sodium valproate 26, 86, 148, 150, 203

Spastic quadriplegia 24, 147

Specificity 14, 134, 224

Speech development 86, 212

Spina bifida 22, 145

Squint 16, 87, 137, 214

Statistics 13, 97, 134, 224

Stepping reflex 84, 211

Stillbirth rate 12, 132

Still's murmur 31, 157

Strabismus 22, 23

Stranger anxiety 7, 125

Strategy meeting 9, 128

Strawberry naevus 39

Sturge- Weber syndrome 39, 110

Subacute sclerosing panencephalitis 15

Subarachnoid haemorrhage 59

Subdural haematoma 59, 185

Subungual fibromas 62, 188

Sudden infant death syndrome 73, 84, 93, 200, 211, 220

Suicide 87, 214, 245

Supervision Order 9, 129

Surfactant 45, 172

Surfactant deficiency 121, 245

Sweat sodium test 80, 208

T

Talipes equinovarus 71, 198

Tall stature 56, 92, 182

Temporal lobe epilepsy 25

Tetralogy of Fallot 29, 76, 77, 104, 125, 154, 203, 205, 229

Tinea capitis 96, 166, 223

Tinea corporis 96, 223

Tinea pedis 96, 224

Toe- walking 105 231

Torsion of the testis 20

Toxoplasma 72, 199

Transposition of the great arteries 30, 32, 155, 157, 228, 229

Treacher- Collins syndrome 17

Trendelenberg test 118, 242

Tuberous sclerosis 18, 19, 62, 139, 140, 188

U

Umbilical hernia 111, 236

Unconjugated hyperbilirubinaemia 42, 83, 168, 210

Undescended testes 108, 113, 234

Urinary tract infection 55, 181, 247

V

Venous hum 31, 157

Ventricular septal defect 29, 75, 104, 125, 146, 153, 230

Vesico -ureteric reflux 55, 114, 239

Vigabatrin 26

Viral hepatitis 44

Visual impairment 16, 47, 136

Visual loss 16, 136

Vitamin D deficiency 115, 240

Von Spitz sign 36, 162

W

Whooping cough 11, 32, 56, 131, 158, 183

William's syndrome 35, 161

Wilm's tumour 51, 52, 177, 179

Wilson's disease 43, 169

Wolff- Parkinson- White Syndrome 11

X

X linked recessive 73, 199

Y

Z

Zoster immunoglobulin 72, 84

www.ingramcontent.com/pod-product-compliance
Lightning Source LLC
Chambersburg PA
CBHW051633170526
45167CB00001B/179